AF696343

DESCARTES AND THE PUZZLE OF SENSORY REPRESENTATION

Descartes and the Puzzle of Sensory Representation

RAFFAELLA DE ROSA

OXFORD
UNIVERSITY PRESS

OXFORD
UNIVERSITY PRESS

Great Clarendon Street, Oxford OX2 6DP

Oxford University Press is a department of the University of Oxford.
It furthers the University's objective of excellence in research, scholarship,
and education by publishing worldwide in

Oxford New York

Auckland Cape Town Dar es Salaam Hong Kong Karachi
Kuala Lumpur Madrid Melbourne Mexico City Nairobi
New Delhi Shanghai Taipei Toronto

With offices in

Argentina Austria Brazil Chile Czech Republic France Greece
Guatemala Hungary Italy Japan Poland Portugal Singapore
South Korea Switzerland Thailand Turkey Ukraine Vietnam

Oxford is a registered trade mark of Oxford University Press
in the UK and in certain other countries

Published in the United States
by Oxford University Press Inc., New York

© Raffaella De Rosa 2010

The moral rights of the author have been asserted
Database right Oxford University Press (maker)

First published 2010

All rights reserved. No part of this publication may be reproduced,
stored in a retrieval system, or transmitted, in any form or by any means,
without the prior permission in writing of Oxford University Press,
or as expressly permitted by law, or under terms agreed with the appropriate
reprographics rights organization. Enquiries concerning reproduction
outside the scope of the above should be sent to the Rights Department,
Oxford University Press, at the address above

You must not circulate this book in any other binding or cover
and you must impose the same condition on any acquirer

British Library Cataloguing in Publication Data
Data available

Library of Congress Cataloging in Publication Data
Data available

Typeset by SPI Publisher Services, Pondicherry, India
Printed in Great Britain
on acid-free paper by the
MPG Books Group, Bodmin and King's Lynn

ISBN 978–0–19–957037–9

To my parents, Meri and Raffaele De Rosa

Contents

Preface

So much has been written on Descartes, including his theory of mind and ideas. Why then a new book on the topic? The short answer is that no systematic account of Descartes' theory of sensory representation is currently available. In particular, there is no systematic study that explains how the complexity and richness of Descartes' views on sensory representation is compatible with (what I will argue to be) his claim that sensory ideas misrepresent their objects in normal circumstances. This book is an ambitious attempt to fill this gap. It provides a novel account of the representationality of Cartesian sensations that is critical of, and different from, all other extant accounts.

The longer answer is that a systematic account of Descartes' views of sensory representation is necessary both to help overthrow long-standing misconceptions of his account of sensation and to highlight his legacy and timeless contribution to still open-ended philosophical questions. Descartes gave a fairly elaborate account of the workings of the human sensory faculty. However, both seventeenth-century scholars and contemporary philosophers of mind hold that Descartes' rampant rationalism prevented him from assigning any genuine cognitive role to the senses. Sensations are impressionistic modes of the mind that are at best cognitively useless (since they carry no information) and at worst cognitively dangerous (since they lead to error). Because of this widespread view, only a few have attempted to argue that Cartesian sensations are representational. Even among those who agree that Cartesian sensations are representational, only a few try to provide an explicit account of what makes sensations representational. The aim of the present book is to discredit once and for all the view that Cartesian sensations lack representationality by providing a clear and detailed account of what makes them representational. To this end, I defend a reading of Cartesian sensations that assigns a cognitive role to them which is proprietary to the senses (although not wholly independent of the intellect) and consistent with the Cartesian claim that sensations are modes of the mind–body union. My claim is that Descartes held a hybrid theory of sensory representation that combines elements of his internalism, rationalism and nativism with a causal account of sensation. This hybrid theory attributes a positive role to the senses within the cognitive architecture of the Cartesian mind and, hence, contributes to their rehabilitation within Descartes' overall rationalist philosophy. Moreover, in explaining Descartes' view that sensations have qualitative character without lacking representationality and his view of the mechanisms of sensory misrepresentation, this book addresses questions which are still of great interest in the contemporary philosophy of mind and cognitive science (for example, how is it possible for any theory of mental content to explain misrepresentation? Are there *qualia*?).

So, the book, in addition to intending to contribute to Descartes scholarship, also raises broader issues about the role of sensations (*qua* modes of the mind–body union) within the cognitive architecture of the Cartesian mind and about the problem of mental representation and misrepresentation. As a result, the book aims to draw the attention of both seventeenth-century scholars and philosophers of mind with an interest in early modern theories of mental representation.

A few words about the scope and underlying strategy of the book are in order. Descartes includes in the sensory perceptions belonging to the embodied mind not only sensations of color, taste and sound (i.e., of so-called secondary qualities) but also bodily sensations such as hunger, thirst and pain and emotions such as fear and love. To focus this study, my book is dedicated only to the first class of sensory perceptions and will have little to say about the latter two. Moreover, the book focuses on those *mental* mechanisms that explain the representationality of sensations of secondary qualities rather than on an analysis of the metaphysics of these qualities. Although these issues are related, in Descartes' case the question of the intentionality of sensation cannot be solved by providing an account of the correct metaphysics of secondary qualities and, so, the two questions are largely independent.

Finally, the book combines an historical analysis of Descartes' conception of sensory representation with a more philosophical approach that relates Descartes' views to contemporary accounts of mental representation. As a result, I will often employ contemporary concepts and terminology in my discussion of Descartes' views on ideas. Some Descartes scholars may be suspicious of this approach, but my strategy is to use contemporary terminology as a neutral tool to understand Descartes' own views. The underlying conviction is that historical figures are part of an everlasting debate over some basic philosophical problems whose intrinsic interest still vexes us. On the one hand, contemporary theoretical tools may help illuminate issues discussed by Descartes; on the other, the contemporary reader may re-discover that Descartes' discussion of mental representation is more relevant to contemporary issues than initially expected.

The end result is a book that offers a novel account of the representationality of Cartesian sensations; provides a panoramic overview, and critical assessment, of the scholarly literature on this issue; and places Descartes' theory of sensation in the central position it deserves among the philosophical and scientific investigations of the workings of the human mind.

Raffaella De Rosa

Guttenberg, New Jersey
March 2009

Acknowledgments

In 2004, I published "Descartes on Sensory Misrepresentation: the Case of Materially False Ideas" (*History of Philosophy Quarterly*, 21, 3, 2004, pp. 261–280), on the rather specialized topic of how to make sense of materially false ideas. Later on, my interest shifted towards the more general question of the psychological and causal mechanisms that, according to Descartes, underpin sensory representation. Since that first article, my views have evolved into a more substantial explanation of Descartes' views on sensations. And the present book offers a positive account of sensory representation and misrepresentation that differs significantly from the one outlined in the earlier article. The difficulties I faced in trying to defend my earlier claim that the initial representationality of Cartesian sensations is to be explained in virtue of a causal connection between the mind and the environment prompted me to examine alternative positions on Cartesian sensations in the current literature. The discussion and critical evaluation of these positions take up the polemical part of the present book and lead up to my own novel account.

In the last five years, I presented both earlier versions of various chapters of the book, and different papers whose content was later incorporated in the book, at different colloquia and conferences at Harvard University, CUNY Graduate Center, University of Oslo, University of Istanbul, Bogaziçi University, Dalhousie University, Lewis and Clark College, University of Zagreb, Northwestern University, University of Siena. I would like to thank the various audiences of these sessions. I also owe special thanks to all my colleagues in the New York metropolitan area who either regularly or occasionally attend the NY/NJ Workshop in Early Modern Philosophy. Two sessions (one on the teleology of Cartesian sensations, with Alison Simmons and Daniel Garber on the panel, and one on the discussion of causal accounts of Cartesian sensations) were organized and gave me a great opportunity to present some of the views defended in the book and receive excellent feedback.

Over the years, many colleagues (possibly more than I can remember) have given me comments on the book material either in a written or spoken format (or both). Sean Greenberg (for always offering prompt, insightful and challenging comments on the book material at various stages); Andrew Pessin and Andrew Chignell (for our conversations on these topics and for giving me the opportunity to read their work on Cartesian sensations when it was still unpublished); Richard Field (to whom I owe an intense and very helpful correspondence over our different readings of the representationality of ideas of sense); Alison Simmons and Tad Schmaltz (for their generosity and open-mind in hearing my criticisms of their views and raising challenging questions for my own views); Alan Gabbey (for providing helpful written comments on what is now Chapter 3 in the book); Lilli Alanen (for asking challenging questions about my reading of the teleology of Cartesian sensations); Michael Della Rocca and Alan Nelson (for providing very useful written comments on what is now Chapter 4 in the book); Ernest Lepore (for many stimulating conversations on book related topics); and the referees of the book for OUP (for their generous and insightful comments). Three people, however, deserve extra-special thanks. Daniel Garber, for inviting me to present some of the book material in his graduate seminar "Cartesian Dualism and the 17th Century Materialism" at Princeton University in the Spring of 2007, and for providing very helpful feedback on the manuscript on many different occasions during the semester I spent at Princeton as a visiting assistant professor; Martha Bolton, for her numerous discussions of the topics of the book and for being an important influence on my work in Descartes' philosophy of mind; and Thomas Vinci, whom I first met at a Meeting of the Atlantic Canada Seminar in Early Modern Philosophy in 2005 and who has been a terrific colleague ever since. He encouraged my work, engaged in numerous philosophical discussions with me and provided some of the most insightful criticisms of my view. To all of you: Thank you for all your precious feedback; I can only hope to have responded in some adequate way to your comments.

I also would like to thank Peter Momtchiloff from OUP for his generous assistance throughout the publication process; Sara Barnes for copyediting; and Michael Johnson for compiling the index.

On a more personal note, I want to thank my son, Matteo, for keeping me focused on completing the manuscript before his birth and for making the year 2008 an extraordinarily good one. I am very much indebted to Carmen Suarez, who brought happiness and love to Matteo during the hours I spent revising the manuscript. Thanks to my loving parents, Meri and Raffaele De Rosa, for their unqualified support; to my father, Raffaele de Rosa, for his painting "Il Castello di Podenzana"; and to my younger brother, Nicola, for his ability to make me always laugh about the hardship of writing philosophy. Last, but not least, I want to thank Ernie Lepore for his love and support and for sharing with me the bliss and hardship of parenthood.

Crucial to my completion of the manuscript were three different periods of research free of teaching duties. These periods were made possible by an NEH Summer Stipend in the Summer of 2006; a sabbatical leave in the Fall of 2006 and a family leave in the Spring of 2008 (both from Rutgers Newark).

Descartes' descriptivist account of ideas in Chapter 1 is reproduced from my article "Descartes on Sensory Misrepresentation: the Case of Materially False Ideas," *History of Philosophy Quarterly*, 21, 3, 2004, pp. 261–280. (There I call Descartes' account a "presentational account.") The passage is on pp. 262–263 and is reprinted with kind permission of the editor of *History of Philosophy Quarterly*. I am grateful also to Wiley-Blackwell for letting me re-use materials from my article "The Myth of Cartesian Qualia," *Pacific Philosophical Quarterly*, 88, 2, 2007, pp. 181–207 in Chapter 2. Some portions of Chapter 4 are reproduced from my article "A Teleological Account of Cartesian Sensations?" *Synthese*, 156, 2007, pp. 317–342 with kind permission of Springer Science and Business Media.

Abbreviations

ABBREVIATIONS FOR CITED PRIMARY TEXTS

AT	Descartes, R. (1964–74). *Oeuvres de Descartes.* Ed. C. Adam and P. Tannery, vols. I–XI, Paris, Libraire Philosophique J. Vrin, cited by volume and page.
CSM	Descartes, R. (1984–85). *The Philosophical Writings of Descartes.* Ed. and trans. J. Cottingham, R. Stoothoff and D. Murdoch, Volumes I–II, Cambridge, Cambridge University Press, cited by volume and page.
CSMK	Descartes, R. (1991). *The Philosophical Writings of Descartes. The Correspondence.* Ed. and trans. J. Cottingham, R. Stoothoff, D. Murdoch and A. Kenny, Volume III, Cambridge, Cambridge University Press, cited by volume and page.
S	Malebranche, N. (1997). *The Search After Truth.* Ed. and trans. T. M. Lennon and P. J. Olscamp. Cambridge, Cambridge University Press, cited by book, chapter and page.

Frequently used abbreviations

DA Descriptivist account of ideas
CA Causal account of ideas
TA Teleofunctional account of ideas

Overview

The aim of this overview is to introduce the reader to the problem of sensory representation in Descartes scholarship and outline my argumentative strategies for solving it. First, I will explain why the phenomenon of sensory representation constitutes an exegetical and theoretical problem for Descartes and why it necessitates a solution. Then, I will describe solutions that unfold from the accounts of Cartesian sensations currently available; I will briefly explain why I disagree with these accounts and solutions, and lastly, I will advertise the position I will defend. The detailed arguments for these various claims are in the ensuing chapters.

THE EXEGETICAL AND THEORETICAL PROBLEM: THE PUZZLE OF SENSORY REPRESENTATION

According to Descartes, the senses misrepresent the material world and its properties in normal circumstances. If I look at the sun and represent it as a flat small yellow disk in the sky, I misrepresent it. Paradigm cases of sensory misrepresentation include ideas of so-called "secondary qualities" such as color and taste, since these represent their objects (i.e., bodies) as other than they are (i.e., as resembling the felt sensation of color and taste). The idea of red represents bodies as red. But since bodies do not instantiate the property of redness as we experience it, the idea of red misrepresents the properties of the material world. Descartes calls ideas of secondary qualities "materially false" in Meditation Three and in the Fourth Set of Replies and continues to regard them as misrepresentations of the material world in all subsequent works.

Despite this *leitmotiv* in his writings, Descartes never explicitly accounted for the psychological and causal mechanisms underlying sensory misrepresentation.

What this account may be in Descartes' philosophy of mind is particularly pressing since his general theory of ideas makes it impossible for an idea to misrepresent its object. Descartes holds what I will call a "descriptivist account of ideas" (DA), according to which, the object of an idea is determined by an identifying description expressed by the mode of presentation of the idea. For an idea to be an idea of *x*, then, it cannot represent *x* as other than *x* is, on pain of not being an idea of *x*. In light of this general account of ideas, Descartes' claim that sensory ideas are misrepresentations of their objects in normal circumstances is particularly puzzling. How can a sensory idea be a representation of *x* and yet misrepresent *x* at the same time? It follows from DA that either a sensory idea represents its object correctly or, if not, it is not the idea of that object.

This puzzle splinters into three different, albeit related, questions. First, what does Descartes mean by the claim that sensory ideas misrepresent their objects or represent their objects as other than they are? Does he mean to imply that an idea can refer to an object *x* but present an object *y* to the mind? Or does he mean something more subtle? Does, perhaps, his claim concern his view that sensory ideas are instances of obscure and confused thoughts? The texts do not clearly answer these questions and, so, even establishing what Descartes meant by claiming that sensory ideas are misrepresentations will require substantial exegesis.

Second, does Descartes' account of sensory representation deviate from his general account of ideas, *viz.*, DA? One may argue that since DA applies only to intellectual ideas, and sensory ideas differ from intellectual ones insofar as they are the by-product of the mind–body union, sensory ideas also exhibit different mechanisms of representation. Or, did Descartes hold an account of sensory representation consistent with DA despite the fact that sensory ideas are modes of the mind–body union? These questions raise the broader issue of the relation between the senses and the intellect within the cognitive architecture of the Cartesian mind.

Third, whether or not Descartes held a unitary theory of mental representation, what mechanisms explain why the idea of red (for example) represents a bodily configuration as other than it actually is? Any account that aims at explaining Descartes' theory of sensory representation ought to include an explanation of how sensory ideas are misrepresentations of their objects in normal circumstances.

AIM AND SCOPE

The present book is an ambitious (albeit limited) attempt to reconstruct the account of sensory representation and misrepresentation that Descartes failed (for whatever reason) to bequeath us by addressing the various questions listed above. I will focus on ideas of secondary qualities (*viz.*, color, taste, sound) and tender a novel interpretation of Descartes' account of these ideas that provides an explanation of the phenomenon of sensory misrepresentation. Before presenting my account, I will discuss and criticize other currently available proposals of how either to dodge or to solve the puzzle. The end result is, then, a systematic overview, and critical evaluation, of the current literature on this topic that culminates with an alternative account of Descartes' views on sensory representation and misrepresentation.

Possible solutions to Descartes' puzzle of misrepresentation can be identified in the literature in various books and articles discussing either Descartes' notion of material falsity or his causal principles or sensation in general.[1] Since the argumentative strategies underlying these solutions stem, by and large, from different ways of understanding Descartes' views on sensations, let me preface the introduction of these solutions with an overview of currently available views on Cartesian sensations.

THE PRESENT STATUS OF THE LITERATURE ON CARTESIAN SENSATIONS

The literature on Cartesian sensations divides into two main strands, the non-representationalist and the representationalist strand.[2] According to

[1] I should clarify that not all the arguments that I will present as possible argumentative strategies to solve the puzzle of misrepresentation were explicitly couched in these terms. The exception is Margaret Wilson, who (to my knowledge) was the first to bring this exegetical problem to our attention and to offer an explicit solution to it.

[2] For a similar taxonomy see Simmons (1999).

the non-representationalist reading, Cartesian sensations lack intrinsic intentionality.[3] Sensations present themselves as non-relational and purely qualitative features of experience, that is, they are what in the contemporary literature are called *qualia.* Accordingly, Descartes' view would be that in perceiving a color such as red, one is merely experiencing the subjective feel of redness rather than perceiving (or seeming to perceive) a bodily surface as red. The intentionality that sensations exhibit is, then, only inherited from some implicit judgment we make. Despite the fact that this reading has been defended only by a few scholars in print,[4] it is still the standard view among most early modern philosophy scholars and contemporary philosophers of mind.

Scholars who defend a representationalist reading divide into two camps, although they all share the view that sensations are *intrinsically* representational, that is, they represent what they do independently of, and prior to, any act of judgment. According to some scholars, Cartesian sensations only apparently represent something real.[5] According to others, Cartesian sensations not only apparently but also actually represent something real.[6] More precisely, sensations are obscure and confused representations of modes of *res extensa.*

In this book, I will discuss the possible solutions to the puzzle of misrepresentation that stem from both the non-representationalist reading and the representationalist view that sensations are obscure and confused representations of modes of *res extensa.*[7]

[3] I use "representationality" interchangeably with "intentionality." The property of intentionality is the property ideas have of representing, or seeming to represent, something outside themselves. Although Descartes' notion of representation is essentially a notion of *presentation*, sensory ideas are modes of presentation of objects that are taken to exist outside the mind. I will argue for this interpretation of Descartes more extensively in Chapters 1 and 2 below.

[4] See, for example, Alanen (1994), (2003), Vinci (1998), MacKenzie (1990) and Wilson (1978). According to Wilson (1978), Descartes held this view in the *Principles* but not in earlier writings. Vinci also argues that this is Descartes' explicit position on sensations in the *Principles.* See Vinci (1998), chapter seven.

[5] See, for example, Normore (1986) and Wilson (1978). According to Wilson (1978), Descartes held this view in the *Meditations* but abandoned it in the *Principles* in favor of a non-representationalist view.

[6] See, for example, Bolton (1986); Schmaltz (1992); Simmons (1999) and Wilson (1990).

[7] As we shall see below, I believe that the view that Cartesian sensations only *seem* to represent something real without actually representing it is not tenable. Moreover, it has been argued that since Cartesian sensations, clearly understood, are nothing but *qualia*, ideas of

FIRST STRATEGY: NON-REPRESENTATIONALIST SOLUTIONS

According to scholars who defend a non-representationalist reading of Cartesian sensations, the puzzle is a red herring. Since the puzzle is generated by the claim that sensations are representational, the denial of that claim implies the rejection of the puzzle. The tenability of this strategy depends, then, on whether we can deny that Descartes attributed intrinsic intentionality to sensations and establish instead that he treated them as purely decorative states of the mind (or *qualia*). Despite various differences among proponents of a non-representationalist reading, they all invoke either arguments intended to show that Descartes could not possibly hold the view that sensations are representational or some specific texts intended to provide evidence that this is so. However, neither the arguments nor the texts establish that Descartes denied that sensations are representational and, hence, this argumentative strategy is untenable. Cartesian sensations are representational. So, the puzzle of sensory misrepresentation requires an explanation.

SECOND SET OF STRATEGIES: EXTERNALIST SOLUTIONS

Among scholars who defend the representationalist view that ideas of secondary qualities are obscure and confused representations of corporeal reality, quite a few (more or less explicitly) have opted for a causal reading of the representationality of sensations. The argument is simple. Descartes' DA renders it impossible to explain the notion of sensory misrepresentation; however, Descartes is committed to the view that ideas of sense represent their objects as other than they are; it is possible

sense are representations of *qualia* or modes of the mind. See, for example, Nelson (1996) and Field (1993). Thomas Vinci also maintains that this is what underlies Descartes' notion of material falsity in Meditation Three. See Vinci (1998), pp. 180–194. But as long as these views assume that sensations *per se* lack any intrinsic intentionality, I consider them variants of the non-representationalist interpretation. See Chapter 2 below.

to explain this view *only if* we attribute to Descartes a causal account of the representationality of sensory ideas, according to which ideas represent their correct objects in virtue of a regular causal connection with them. Therefore, Descartes does not subscribe to DA for sensory ideas. He holds a causal account instead.

The main advantage of, and motivation for, this reading consists in explaining the phenomenon of sensory misrepresentation. Since a sensory idea represents its object in virtue of a causal relation and independently of how the object is presented to the mind, the object presented to the mind may differ from the object the idea actually refers to. So, an explanation is provided for why a sensory idea represents its correct object as other than it actually is. However, I will argue that the allure of this reading is only apparent for several reasons. First of all, it is possible to read the phrase "sensory ideas represent their objects as other than they are" in an alternative way consistent with DA. Secondly, not only do causal accounts fail to explain the representationality of sensations, but they also fail to have their most advertised advantage, that is, that of solving the puzzle of misrepresentation. Finally, the textual evidence invoked in their support (for example, the passages where Descartes insists that sensations are modes of the mind–body union and that bodies are causally responsible for our having sensory ideas) does not incontrovertibly support this reading.

Another externalist reading of Descartes' account of the representationality of sensations is teleofunctional. According to this view, Cartesian sensations are regularly caused by the bodies that they represent because of their functional/biological role of securing the survival of the mind–body union. Despite the fact that a teleofunctional account builds on a causal one, it does not share its main motivation, that is, that of solving the puzzle of misrepresentation. On the contrary, one of the claimed advantages of this account is that, once we understand that the proper function of the senses differs from that of the intellect, we also understand that ideas of sense are not misrepresentations of their objects but represent them exactly as they should. Roughly, the idea is that since the role of the senses consists in preserving the mind–body union, sensory ideas represent the external world as-it-is-in-relation-to-the-mind (as opposed as it is in itself). And in as long as they do this successfully, they are correct representations of their objects or "materially true." So, the puzzle of misrepresentation would be generated by a false expectation of what sensory ideas represent. Once this expectation is dissolved, so is the puzzle.

Unfortunately, a teleofunctional account is untenable. Aside from the fact that Descartes never claimed that sensations are "materially true" and that the texts do not uncontroversially support a teleofunctional reading, other difficulties confound this proposal. First, the theoretical costs of having Cartesian sensations come out "materially true" are too high to be negotiated for its benefits. A teleofunctional account of the representationality of sensations, in fact, introduces more theoretical problems than it solves (either for Descartes or in general). Second, it is not even clear that a teleofunctional account has the benefits it claims to have, for, even on this account, sensory ideas turn out to be misrepresentations of their objects.

THIRD SET OF STRATEGIES: PURELY INTERNALIST SOLUTIONS

Internalist readings aren't the most popular ones (non-representationalist and the causal accounts being by far the most commonly endorsed) but a few can be identified in the literature. Here are their highlights in contrast with externalist accounts. According to internalist readings, by and large, the attribution of a causal theory of sensory representation to Descartes is not forced on us by his account of sensory misrepresentation because we can interpret Descartes' claim that sensory ideas represent their objects as other than they are in a way compatible with DA. Rather than reading the phrase "sensory ideas represent their objects as other than they are" as implying that these ideas refer to one object but present another to the mind, advocates of internalist accounts suggest that it ought to be read as implying that sensory ideas contain an obscure and confused description of the correct object of thought. The claim is that the obscure and confused presentation of the object of thought already contains, so to speak, the correct object even if this object is not immediately evident to the subject. If this is a plausible reading (as I think it is), then it follows that the texts (*contra* what advocates of causal accounts want to say) do not force us to attribute to Descartes a theory of sensory representation that wreaks havoc with DA.

It still remains to be explained – even along the lines of DA – how an idea can represent its correct object if this object is not immediately evident to the subject, or, *mutatis mutandis*, how an idea can be an obscure and confused representation of its correct object. The puzzle of misrepresentation does not go away in virtue of endorsing a reading of Descartes' claim that sensations misrepresent their objects along the lines of DA. I have identified at least two different answers to this question in the current literature. Either the fact that sensory ideas represent their correct objects obscurely is explained by virtue of an intrinsic and primitive feature of such ideas; or by virtue of the presence of a semi-hidden intelligible content in the sensory content.

Although I am sympathetic to an overall internalist approach, I find the currently available internalist accounts insufficient to fully explain *sensory* representation and misrepresentation. One of these theories provides no internalist *account* of the representationality of sensation since it concludes that the relation of sensory representation is a primitive (and, hence, inexplicable) notion. The other account provides a persuasive internalist explanation of the representationality of Cartesian sensations (*viz.*, in virtue of some hidden intelligible content) but fails to distinguish between *sensory* and intellectual representation. I conclude that despite their advantages, purely internalist theories fail to provide a completely satisfactory explanation of the mechanisms of sensory representation and misrepresentation.

A DESCRIPTIVIST-CAUSAL ACCOUNT

I will defend a *qualified* internalist account that I call "descriptivist-causal." I agree with internalist readings that it is possible to interpret Descartes' claim that sensory ideas represent their objects as other than they are in a way consistent with DA. In particular, I agree that the representationality of sensations is to be explained in virtue of an intelligible content that is latently present in sensory content and only minimally accessed by the subject. The quasi-hidden presence of this intelligible content (partly) explains why sensory ideas represent their correct objects obscurely and confusedly since it allows the idea to represent what it does even if the subject is not fully aware of *what* the object being represented is.

I disagree that consideration of purely internal features of sensory ideas are sufficient to provide a fully satisfactory explanation of sensory representation. My view is that the role of the mind's causal interaction with the environment must be incorporated in Descartes' overall internalist account in order to account for the distinguishing features of sensory representation. First, I defend the suggestion that the *representationality* of sensations is due to the presence of a quasi-hidden intelligible content in light of Descartes' doctrines of innate ideas and his view that all mental acts are operations of the intellect. Second, I argue that Descartes' claim that in having sensory ideas the mind is *affected* by different variations in bodies amounts to his claim that a causal connection with bodies is responsible for the *phenomenological* aspect of sensory ideas. This aspect of Descartes' account has been ignored by purely internalist accounts and erroneously explained by proponents of externalist accounts.

On my view, the presentational content of sensory ideas is determined by two factors.[8] On the one hand, the causal connection of the mind with external bodies accounts for the phenomenology typically constitutive of sensory ideas. On the other hand, the object being presented to the mind is not determined by the causal connection itself but rather by a latent conceptual description of the object. Once this is clarified, the mechanisms of sensory representation and misrepresentations are easily explained. Descartes relates the notion of sensory misrepresentation to that of obscurity and confusion throughout his whole body of work. What makes sensory ideas obscure and confused, on my account, is the natural confusion of the latent conceptualization of the object of thought (coming from the mind) and the phenomenological content (coming from the causal interaction with particular types of configurations of matter). Consequently, sensory ideas represent their objects as other than they are because their presentational content contains not only the identifying description of the object but also the qualitative content derived from the interaction with the environment.

My explanation of sensory misrepresentation neither requires denying the textually grounded thesis that sensations are representational nor denying that Descartes held a unitary theory of mental representation nor ignoring (or misinterpreting) Descartes' views that sensations are modes of the mind–body union. The missing account of sensory representation and misrepresentation that Descartes failed to bequeath

[8] I will clarify the notion of presentational content in Chapter 1 below. As it will become clear in Chapters 5 and 6, on my view, these two components of the presentational content of sensory ideas are inseparable (or fused together) in the infantile mind.

us is then reconstructed in a way that is not only compatible with Descartes' texts and the basic tenets of his philosophy of mind but also theoretically plausible.

THE ROAD AHEAD

Chapter 1 argues that Descartes held a descriptivist account of ideas (DA) and explains in more detail why Descartes' views on the sensory representation of secondary qualities constitute a puzzle in light of DA. This chapter presents the textual evidence and argumentations that lead up to the theoretical issues discussed in the following chapters.

Chapter 2 refutes the widespread non-representationalist reading of Cartesian sensations and, hence, undermines one way of accommodating the puzzle of misrepresentation. This chapter occupies a central place in the book because it establishes that Descartes held that sensations are representational.

Chapters 3 and 4 present and criticize the attempts to deal with the puzzle of misrepresentation that stem from externalist readings of the representationality of sensations. In Chapter 3, I challenge causal readings. (Although most of my arguments against causal accounts of Cartesian sensations are to be found in this chapter, my critical discussion of the textual evidence offered in their support will be found in Chapter 5.) In Chapter 4, I criticize teleofunctional accounts of Cartesian sensations. Although this type of account builds on a causal account, it suffers from difficulties of its own and merits separate attention.

Chapter 5 discusses purely internalist views and contains a defense of my own descriptivist-causal account of Cartesian sensations together with its solution to the puzzle of sensory misrepresentation.

Chapter 6 addresses various objections to my descriptivist-causal account. A brief conclusion follows with a summary of the advantages of my account over those surveyed and discussed in the book.

1

Descartes' Account of Ideas and the Puzzle of Sensory Representation

I begin with a presentation of Descartes' general account of ideas and defend my claim that Descartes held a descriptivist account (DA) (1.1–1.2). Then, I proceed to explain why Descartes' views on sensations of secondary qualities constitute a puzzle in light of DA and why it is necessary to address this puzzle (1.3–1.4). I will also introduce some terminology that will be used throughout the book and conclude with some preliminary caveats (1.5–1.6).

1.1 DESCARTES ON IDEAS

In order to appreciate the nature of the puzzle generated by sensations of secondary qualities, we must begin with an outline of the basic tenets of Descartes' theory of ideas. In Meditation Three, Descartes defines *ideas* as those modes of the mind that are "as it were the images of things" ("*Tanquam rerum images*" CSM II 25; AT VII 37), that is, as modes of the mind that *represent* things.[1] But the notion of representation is a theoretically complex one. And a theory of ideas ought to clarify the

[1] As is clear from the exchange with Hobbes (especially CSM II 126–128; AT VII 179–181), by saying that ideas are like images of things Descartes does not imply that ideas are mental pictures or "images depicted in the corporeal imagination" (CSM II 127; AT VII 181). Rather, according to Descartes, ideas are images insofar as they are representational. On this see, for example, Wilson (1978), p. 102. The French translation of the Latin "*Et quia nullae ideae nisi tanquam rerum esse possunt*" (AT VII 44) is: "et d'autant que, les idées étant comme des images, il n'y en peut avoir aucune qui ne nous semble représenter quelque chose" (since ideas are like images, there cannot be any idea that does not seem to represent something). See also the definition of ideas in Axiom II of Second Set of Replies, CSM II 113; AT VII 160–161.

sense in which ideas are representations. In Descartes' case, representation is primarily *presentation* of an object to the mind insofar as *representing something* consists in putting the mind in *cognitive* contact with extra-mental reality.[2] Using a more contemporary terminology, we can say that, according to Descartes, the representational content of the idea is not exhausted, or individuated by, the referent of the idea. Rather, ideas are individuated by the way in which the object is presented to the mind, i.e., by (what I will call) the "*mode of presentation*" of the object.[3] Although this is not Descartes' wording, it helps to understand and explain his claim that ideas are individuated by *their objective reality*. Descartes' views on objective reality have generated numerous and complex discussions in the secondary literature and I cannot possibly do justice to all of them in this context. Instead I will present my own reading of this notion and support it textually.

As is well known, according to Descartes, "ideas" can be taken either *materialiter* (materially) to designate an operation of the mind and, in this sense, all ideas are the same; or *objective* (objectively) to designate the object of thought (i.e., the thing represented) and, in this sense, all ideas are different. In Meditation Three, Descartes writes:

> In so far as the ideas are <considered> simply <as> modes of thought, there is no recognizable inequality among them: they all appear to come from within me in the same fashion. But in so far as different ideas <are considered as images which> represent different things, it is clear that they differ widely. Undoubtedly, the ideas which represent substances to me amount to something more and, so to speak, contain within themselves more objective reality than the ideas which merely represent modes or accidents. Again, the idea that gives me understanding of a supreme God [. . .] certainly has in it more objective reality than the ideas that represent finite substances. (CSM II 27–8; AT VII 40)

[2] On this, see, for example, Chappell (1986) and Wilson (1978), chapter three.

[3] The terminology goes back to Gottlob Frege but it was Margaret Wilson who first distinguished between a presentational and referential content in Descartes' account of ideas in her Wilson (1990). For the time being, I will leave aside the discussion of the relation between the presentational content and referential content. Obviously, it is not very interesting to say that ideas are individuated more finely than by the objects they refer to since everybody concedes that we can have different descriptions of the same object. The interesting issue is whether or not the referent of ideas is considered to be determined by these modes of presentation. And the question of what view Descartes may have held on this issue will be addressed abundantly below.

Ideas are then individuated by their objective reality, that is, by the objects that they represent to the minds. However, the crucial question remains: how are we to understand the notion of "the object of thought"?

The phrase "the object of thought" is itself ambiguous. It can mean at least three different things: (1) the object that exists in the mind and of which the mind thinks (i.e., a mental object); or (2) the object that seems to exist outside the mind and of which the mind thinks; or (3) the object that actually exists outside the mind and of which the mind thinks.[4] According to (1), "the object that is thought of" is the idea itself and, consequently, objectively taken ideas are distinct from formally taken ideas. The former are the content of the latter. According to (2), the object that is thought of is the external object (whether it exists or not) represented by the idea. Ideas are acts of thought having representational content rather than being the representational content of those acts.[5] Notice that both (1) and (2) imply a presentational account of ideas because on both accounts the identity of the idea does not depend on the actual existence of the object represented. But (1) and (2) differ insofar as only the latter implies that the mind presents an external object to the mind. Since, however, both (1) and (2) imply a presentational account of ideas, the claim that (2) implies the presentation of an external object ought to be read as follows: the idea presents an external object to the mind in virtue of an internal feature of the idea itself (rather than in virtue of some mind–world relation).

I agree with several commentators that by "idea" Descartes meant "*either* the thought of an object *or* [. . .] the object thought of, but not

[4] For a recent discussion that overlooks these distinctions see Brown (2006), chapter four. In various places, Brown seems to assume that either Descartes is a representational realist who holds (1) or a direct realist who holds (3). See, for example, Brown (2006), pp. 90–94. I believe, as we shall see, that Descartes' position is more nuanced than that.

[5] The debate between Malebranche and Arnauld originates from, and is evidence for, the ambiguity between (1) and (2) in Descartes. On this see Nadler (1989). Nadler labels the views on ideas expressed by (1) and (2) above (respectively) "the object-approach" and "the content-approach" to intentionality. About the latter he writes: "The intentionality [. . .] of the act is indifferent to the existence or non-existence of the object intended by the act. This follows from the fact that the [intentionality] is a function of the act's content, of a non-relational intrinsic feature of the act [. . .]" (Nadler (1989), p. 146).

[. . .] a third thing *between* thought and object,"[6] and, accordingly, that Descartes did not hold (1). But did Descartes hold (2) or (3)? According to (2), *the object that is thought of* is the external object (whether it exists or not) represented by the idea. According to (3), *the object that is thought of* is the actually existing external object to which the mind is relationally connected. There is ample evidence that Descartes held (2) rather than (3).[7]

Descartes discusses (implicitly or explicitly) the notions of objective reality and objective being in many places. In the Second Set of Replies, Descartes writes that "existence is contained in the idea or concept of every single thing, since we cannot conceive of anything except as existing. Possible or contingent existence is contained in the concept of a limited thing [. . .]" (CSM II 117; AT VII 166). And in the First Set of Replies, Descartes insists that "possible existence is contained in the concept of everything that we clearly and distinctly understand" (CSM II 83; AT VII 117) and that "our understanding of [. . .] things [other than God] always involves understanding them as if they were existing things [although] it does not follow that they exist" (CSM II 83; AT VII 117). Since ideas are *of* things in virtue of their objective reality and possible existence is contained in the idea *of* every single (finite) thing, it follows that the notion of objective reality is related to possible existence. And so ideas are individuated by the possibly (rather than actually) existing objects to which they refer. This conclusion is confirmed by Descartes' own definition of what he means by objectively-taken

[6] Ayers (1991), p. 57. For similar views, see, for example, Yolton (1984), Vinci (1998), Cook (1987) and Alanen (2003).

[7] I avoid framing the issue of how to read Descartes' notion of objective being in terms of whether he is a direct or indirect realist. The reason is that I do not find these labels helpful in understanding Descartes' view. Since it is unclear how to understand "direct" and "indirect" realism to begin with, depending on how we define these terms, Descartes could be either a direct or indirect realist. I am well aware that it has been claimed (see for example, Yolton (1984)) that the view of ideas as mental entities is responsible for Cartesian skepticism (or "skepticism of the veil of ideas"); whereas the view of ideas as mental acts directed towards external objects is supposed to block this skepticism. As should be clear from the above, however, I doubt that (2) is better positioned than (1) to avoid (or solve) the problem of skepticism. What I believe is that Descartes thought of ideas as ways of making external objects cognitively accessible to the mind and so, in that respect, he held what today would be called a "representationalist theory of the mind." But holding this view does not necessarily imply being a skeptic or being an indirect realist. This is not the place, however, to discuss these issues.

ideas in the Preface to the *Meditations*. There, Descartes writes that an idea can be taken objectively, "as the thing represented" by an operation of the mind "even if [the thing] is not regarded as existing outside the intellect" (CSM II 7; AT VII 8).

Descartes' exchange with Caterus is particularly relevant in this context. Caterus had requested further clarification of Descartes' notion of the objective being of ideas. He asked: "[. . .] what *is* an idea?" (CSM II 66; AT VII 92). According to Descartes, an idea is "the thing that is thought of, in so far as it has objective being in the intellect" (Ibid.). But, what is this so-called objective being in the intellect? Caterus asks. Caterus' own answer is: "According to what I was taught, this is simply a determination of an act of the intellect by means of an object. And this is merely an extraneous label which adds nothing to the thing itself" (Ibid.). Notice that Caterus' answer implies a criticism of Descartes' definition of objective being because it denies that objective being counts as *being* at all ("Just as 'being seen' is nothing other than an act of vision attributable to myself," Caterus points out, "so 'being thought of', or having objective being in the intellect, is simply a thought of the mind [. . .]" CSM II 67; AT VII 92). The only *being* involved here, according to Caterus, is the being of the object existing outside the mind (the objective being is an extraneous label "which adds nothing to the thing itself"). In other words, as Brown (2006) puts it, Caterus is defending a deflationary reading of the notion of objective being, according to which, it is "simply a way of talking about an idea's (extrinsic) relation to an object."[8]

It is unclear whether Descartes truly understood and satisfactorily addressed Caterus' worries. However, the clarification of the notion of objective being he provided in the First Set of Replies is sufficient for our purposes. Descartes acknowledges that the phrase "object of thought" is ambiguous between (2) and (3). He remarks that Caterus' objection that "objective being is simply a determination of an act of the intellect by means of an object, and this [objective being] is merely an extraneous label which adds nothing to the thing itself" is based on misunderstanding "objective being" as referring to "the thing itself as if it were located outside the intellect" (CSM II 74; AT VII 102). If this

[8] Brown (2006), p. 86.

were the case, Descartes admits, "objective being is certainly an extraneous label" since it does not add anything to the sun existing in the sky ("For example, if anyone asks what happens to the sun through its being objectively in my intellect, the best answer is that nothing happens to it beyond the application of an extraneous label [. . .]" CSM II 74; AT VII 102). But, Descartes goes on:

> [When I was speaking of "objective being in the intellect"] I was speaking of the idea [as opposed to the thing itself existing outside the idea], which is never outside the intellect, and in this sense "objective being" simply means being in the intellect in the way in which objects are normally there. (CSM II 74; AT VII 102)

Then, Descartes illustrates the way in which things are normally in the mind with the example of the sun:

> For example, if anyone asks what happens to the sun through its being objectively in my intellect, the best answer is that [the sun] is in the intellect in the way in which its objects are normally there. By this I mean that the idea of the sun is the sun itself existing in the intellect not of course formally existing, as it does in the heavens, but objectively existing, i.e., in the way in which objects normally are in the intellect. (CSM II 75; AT VII 102)

In the two passages just quoted Descartes clarifies that we ought to understand his claim that "the idea of the sun is the sun itself existing in the intellect" as the claim that the idea of the sun contains the (true) representation of the sun. So, these two passages from Descartes' replies to Caterus confirm that "the object of thought" has to be taken, according to (2) above, as the presentation (or description) of the object rather than the object itself. But the exchange with Caterus also tells us something more about the relation between the presentational content of the idea and its referential content. Descartes is saying here that the idea is not simply a sign for its referent but provides the necessary and sufficient condition for identifying the referent by providing the "true" description of the object ("the idea of the sun is the sun itself existing in the intellect").[9]

[9] Notice that my reading of Descartes' claim that "the idea of the sun is the sun itself existing in the intellect" as the claim that *the idea of the sun contains the true representation of the sun* is my way of denying that Descartes is postulating third things between the mind and external reality, as (1) above implies. Thanks to Thomas Vinci for pointing

Finally, at the beginning of Meditation Six Descartes writes about the idea of the chiliagon:

> [. . .] if I want to think of a chiliagon, although I understand that it is a figure consisting of a thousand sides just as well as I understand the triangle to be a three-sided figure, I do not in the same way imagine the thousand sides [. . .]. It is true that since I am in the habit of imagining something whenever I think of a corporeal thing, I may construct in my mind a confused representation of some figure; but it is clear that this is not a chiliagon. For it differs in no way from the representation I should form if I were thinking of a myriagon, or any figure with many sides. (CSM II 50; AT VII 72)

Descartes writes that an idea is the idea *of* a chiliagon (as opposed to that *of* a myriagon) only if the mind presents to itself (or sees by introspection) a chiliagon which is distinct from a myriagon. This, as Wilson (1990) puts it, "suggests that an idea's referentially representing *a* does depend on the idea's somehow presentationally exhibiting *a*."[10]

In conclusion, all this textual evidence indicates that, according to Descartes, the identity of an idea does not depend on the actual existence of the object represented. An idea is individuated by a *mode of presentation* of the object independently of whether the object exists. Whether ideas are, or have, representational contents, these contents are internally determined as opposed to being relationally, or externally, determined. The representation of the object comes from the mind in the way of a presentation *of* the object.[11] A direct implication of this presentational model of ideas is an internalism (certainly compatible with Descartes' nativism) according to which the representational content of ideas is determined by the ways in which we describe objects rather than in virtue of a mind–world relation.

this out to me. Keeping this in mind is important because this passage could easily be interpreted, and it has been interpreted, as supporting (1) (in as long as Descartes here seems to commit himself to two forms of being, formal and objective being). In my view, Descartes here is simply saying that the idea of the sun contains the identifying properties of its referent, i.e., the sun. That is, according to my reading, Descartes thinks that ideas are directed to real objects not by intentional objects but by their properties. See, on this, Normore (1986) p. 234 and Vinci (1998), pp. 61–64.

[10] See Wilson (1990), reprinted in Wilson (1999), p. 82.

[11] The key issue here is the individuation of ideas. What I am arguing is that they are individuated independently of what they are actually related to and, hence, as we shall see later, that the referential relation is mediated by the presentational content.

1.2 DESCARTES' DESCRIPTIVIST ACCOUNT OF IDEAS (DA)

On the basis of 1.1 above, we can conclude that Descartes held what I will call a "descriptivist account of ideas" (DA) whose basic tenets are:

(DA) (I) Ideas are individuated by their mode of presentation of an object (or objective reality).[12]

(II) The mode of presentation provides an identifying description of the object.

(III) The mode of presentation of an idea determines its object so that the idea refers to whatever corresponds to (or satisfies) its mode of presentation.

(I)–(III), imply (IV): for an idea to be an idea of *n* it cannot represent *n* as other than *n* is (on pain of not being the idea of *n*).[13]

Let me make two general remarks about DA. First, DA is modeled after the clear and distinct ideas of the intellect since, according to Descartes, those are the ideas that present the object to the mind as it actually is. I take (II) to be implied by Descartes' example that *the idea of the sun* is the *sun itself* as it exists in the mind.[14] This is confirmed by Descartes' remark, in his exchange with Arnauld that we must distinguish between

[12] Ideas so individuated are "abstract" ideas in the sense that they represent particular objects and are tokened by different minds or by the same mind at different times. The details of how an abstract idea is related to its tokenings in the mind and the particular objects represented are not relevant in this context. Notice, however, that attributing this view to Descartes does not necessarily commit him to maintain that abstract ideas are abstract objects really distinct from both the finite mind and particular objects, since it is possible to think of abstract ideas as general and innate ways of conceiving of particular things. Despite the presence of a few passages where Descartes seems to suggest that ideas of mathematics are ideas of abstract objects (i.e., "true and immutable essences") which are really distinct from particular objects (for example, CSM II 44–45; AT VII 64), in the *Principles of Philosophy* (among other texts) Descartes seems to hold the view that abstract ideas are innate ways of thinking of particular objects (see, for example, CSM I 211–212; AT VIIIA 26, 27, 28). On this issue, see Bolton (1998), Chappell (1997), Nolan (1997) (1998), Rozemond (2008) and De Rosa and Bueno (2008).

[13] In De Rosa (2004), I called this account of ideas the "presentational account" (see De Rosa (2004), p. 263).

[14] In Meditation Three, Descartes claims that there are two ideas of the sun. There is the sensory idea that misrepresents the sun as something small; and then there is the correct idea of the sun obtained through astronomical reasoning. I am assuming here that Descartes is talking about the latter in the above example.

obscure and confused ideas, on the one hand, and clear and distinct ones, on the other. To Arnauld's objection that the notion of material falsity is inconsistent with DA's tenet that "the idea of *x* is just *x* itself as it exists in the understanding" (our (II) above) Descartes clarifies that this principle only applies to clear and distinct ideas:

> When [Arnauld] says that the idea of cold "is coldness itself in so far as it exists objectively in the intellect" I think we need to make a distinction. For it often happens in the case of confused and obscure ideas – and the ideas of heat and cold fall into this category – that an idea is referred to something other than that of which it is in fact the idea. (CSM II 163; AT VII 233)

In the above passage, (more or less explicitly) Descartes claims that Arnauld's objection (*viz.*, that Descartes' tenet makes it impossible for the idea of cold to be materially false) is ill-founded because the idea of cold is an obscure and confused idea and the tenet applies to ideas that are *not* obscure and confused, that is, (presumably) clear and distinct ideas.

Second, (III) illustrates Descartes' views on reference. It claims that, according to Descartes, the object of the idea (or referent) is the object that, if it existed, would satisfy the description (of the object) contained in the idea.[15] Notice, moreover, that (III) claims that an object is the referent of a certain idea if it *satisfies* (or *corresponds* to) the presentation of the object without implying that there must be a resemblance between the represented object and the actual object.[16]

[15] The idea of God may seem to provide a counterexample to the above definition since in Meditation Three Descartes claims that we could not have the (clear and distinct) idea of God unless God existed and caused it in us. And this may suggest that Descartes offers a causal account of (at least) the idea of God. Besides the fact that the idea of God is unique and, so, the account of its content cannot be extended to the rest of ideas, this is not even what Descartes maintains about the idea of God. Descartes infers that God exists and is the cause of the idea in us *because* of the way in which we clearly and distinctly represent him in our minds.

[16] DA is similar to what Margaret Wilson calls a "presentational account of ideas" (see Wilson (1990), reprinted in Wilson (1999), p. 73). But despite the similarities in formulation, there is a crucial difference between DA and the "presentational account of ideas" that Wilson attributes to Descartes. By attributing this account to Descartes, Wilson attributes to him a theory of ideas that has nothing to do with the referential relation. But, according to DA, Descartes is committed to the view that there must be a correspondence between the presentational and referential contents so that an idea cannot refer to anything other than what the idea presents to the mind. I call my reading of Descartes' theory a "descriptivist account" in order to indicate that Descartes is a "descriptivist" about reference.

1.3 DESCARTES ON SENSORY IDEAS OF SECONDARY QUALITIES: THE TEXTUAL DATA

Descartes didn't always call ideas of secondary qualities "materially false."[17] However, as I will argue, he did hold the consistent view, throughout his whole body of work, that ideas of sense misrepresent the material world insofar as they are obscure and confused ideas that represent their objects (i.e., bodies) as something other than they actually are (that is, as instantiating properties they do not actually instantiate).[18]

In Meditation Three, after claiming that all ideas are "as it were the images of things" (CSM II 25; AT VII 37), Descartes writes that material falsity belongs to ideas of colors, sounds, smell (CSM II 30; AT VII 43) and it occurs when these ideas "represent non-things as things" (CSM II 30; AT VII 43). Here's the famous passage:

> [. . .] material falsity [. . .] occurs in ideas when they represent non-things as things. For example, the ideas I have of heat and cold contain so little clarity and distinctness that they do not enable me to tell whether cold is merely the absence of heat or vice versa, or whether both of them are real qualities, or

[17] As we shall see, Descartes introduces the notion of material falsity in Meditation Three (CSM II 30; AT VII 43). Then, he discusses it again in the Fourth Set of Replies (CSM II 163–164; AT VII 232–235) and in *Conversation with Burman* (CSMK 337; AT V 152).

[18] For a different view, see for example, Wilson (1978), chapter three and Vinci (1998), chapter seven. According to both Wilson (1978) and Vinci (1998), Descartes' views on sensory ideas changed over time. Both claim that in Meditation Three, Descartes still acknowledged that sensations are representational by calling them "materially false." According to Wilson (1978), Descartes is saying that sensations still seem to represent something in the external world but they do not actually represent anything. According to Vinci, Descartes is saying that ideas of sense represent whiteness, redness and so on (which are nothing but sensations) as "quasi-substantial entit[ies] that [are] more than mere mode[s] of substances" (see Vinci (1998), p. 185). But both Wilson (1978) and Vinci (1998) agree that by the time Descartes wrote the *Principles* he had abandoned the view that sensations are representational altogether. I will argue against this reading of the *Principles* in the following chapters. It is worth noticing that Margaret Wilson changed her mind about this issue in Wilson (1990) and argued for a consistency between Descartes' earlier and later texts. Cecilia Wee has argued that Descartes is already changing his definition of material falsity in his replies to Arnauld (see Wee (2006), chapter one). Since I became aware of Wee's book only after I had completed the writing of my book, I was unable to give her views the full consideration that they deserve in this context. For a brief discussion of Wee's views, see De Rosa (2008).

neither is. And since there can be no ideas which are not as it were of things, if it is true that cold is nothing but the absence of heat, the idea which represents it to me as something real and positive deserves to be called false [. . .]. (CSM II 30; AT VII 43–44)

Literally speaking, according to this passage, a materially false idea is an idea that represents a non-entity (i.e., an impossible object) as an entity (i.e., a possible object) or, as Descartes puts it, a privation as something positive.[19] However, the literal meaning cannot be what Descartes had in mind, for several reasons. First, secondary qualities can be either positive or privative properties (if cold is the absence of heat, then heat must be something positive) and, so, at least some ideas of secondary qualities (on the assumption that they represent their objects as something positive) would be materially true. But Descartes suggests that *both* the ideas of heat and cold may fail to represent real qualities ("they do not enable me to tell whether cold is merely the absence of heat or vice versa, or whether both of them are real qualities, or neither is") and, hence, be materially false.[20]

Second, it is at least *prima facie* inconsistent with Descartes' own theory of ideas to claim that an idea "refers" to a certain object (a non-thing) but presents a different one to the mind (a positive thing). If this were the case, then, to use the terminology introduced in the above section, an idea would have a presentational content that is different

[19] The term "thing" here is used loosely to mean anything real whether that is a substance or property of a substance. This is confirmed by the quotation above.

[20] For a similar point see Wilson (1978), p. 109; and Field (1993), p. 317. Moreover, is it even possible for an idea to represent nothing? If Descartes' account of mental representation consists in his theory of objective being, then it is impossible for an idea to represent a complete non-thing. For a literal reading of this passage, see Catherine Wilson (2003), pp. 92–93 and p. 98; Vinci (1998), pp. 184–187; and Wee (2006), chapters one and three. According to Wilson (2003), Descartes introduces ideas of privations to contrast them with the idea of God and as a way of setting up the proof for the existence of God in Meditation Three. I disagree with this way of reading the passage not only for the reasons listed above, but also because Descartes continues the discussion of material falsity with Arnauld and this discussion seems to be about a deeper notion than Wilson (2003) wants it to be. Besides, in reply to Arnauld's pressing criticisms, Descartes would have had the perfect occasion to downplay the notion of material falsity. But he did not. According to Vinci, materially false ideas represent a non-thing (whiteness as it is in itself, that is, a mode of the sensuous mind) as a real quality or quasi-substantial entity. I disagree with this reading because I believe that Descartes is here using "thing" loosely to mean any real property. For my disagreement with Wee, see De Rosa (2008).

from its referential content. But, as we saw above, DA's (I)–(III) imply that an idea of *n* cannot represent *n* as other than *n* is (on pain of not being the idea of *n*). Besides, Descartes' causal principle, in Meditation Three, states that the objective reality of an idea is the mirror image of the formal reality of the object being represented ("[. . .] in order for a given idea to contain such and such objective reality, it must surely derive it from some cause which contains at least as much formal reality as there is objective reality in the idea," CSM II 28–29; AT VII 41). As we shall see in more detail in the following section, Arnauld first pointed out that the notion of material falsity is inconsistent with Descartes' own theory of ideas and related principles. He noted that an idea, according to Descartes' own principles, cannot refer to an object *x* (a non-entity) but exhibit an object *y* (an entity) to the mind:

> [. . .] there cannot be an idea of cold which represents it to me as a positive thing [because] [. . .] what is the idea of cold? It is coldness itself in so far as it exists objectively in the intellect. But if cold is an absence, it cannot exist in the intellect by means of an idea whose objective existence is a positive entity. Therefore, if cold is merely an absence, there cannot be a positive idea of it, and hence there cannot be an idea which is materially false. (CSM II 145; AT VII 206)

Arnauld claims that Descartes' principles make it impossible for him to hold the view that an idea refers to one object but presents a different one to the mind.[21] Each idea is, in and by itself, necessarily true of the object that it exhibits to the mind. He concludes, then, that Cartesian ideas cannot literally represent non-things as things.

Finally, as Arnauld pointed out, "what is the cause of the positive objective being which according to you is responsible for the idea's being materially false? 'The cause is myself', you may answer, 'in so far as I come from nothing.' But in that case, the positive objective being of an idea can come from nothing, which violates the author's most important principles" (CSM II 146; AT VII 207). Arnauld's point is as follows: sensory ideas present something positive to us; but if Descartes holds the view that they come from nothing, then the causal principle is violated (since the objective reality of the idea would be greater than the reality of the object that causes it). But this is a

[21] See Bolton (1986) on this.

possibility Descartes cannot allow for since it would threaten the proof for the existence of God in Meditation Three.

In light of these considerations, I conclude that by calling sensory ideas "materially false" Descartes did not mean to say literally that they represent non-things as things. Instead he meant to say metaphorically that sensory ideas misrepresent their objects or represent their objects as other than they are.

However, a pressing question remains. If sensory ideas are "materially false" in the metaphorical sense of being misrepresentations of their objects, in what sense shall we interpret the phrase *ideas of sense represent their objects as other than they are* vis-à-vis DA's implication that an idea cannot refer to one object and present another to us? There are at least two options here (at least within a representationalist reading of Cartesian sensations).[22] Either Descartes' account of sensory representation wreaks havoc with DA (and, as we shall see in Chapters 3 and 4, this is what externalist readings of Cartesian sensations claim) or it is possible to explain Descartes' notion of sensory misrepresentation in a way that is consistent with DA. In my view, the second option represents Descartes' considered position and I will defend this reading in Chapter 5. For the time being, I only want to note that Descartes begins to provide an answer to this question in his replies to Arnauld's objections.

Descartes *acknowledges* Arnauld's point that the idea of cold cannot represent cold as other than it actually is:

> [. . .] my critic asks what the idea of cold, which I described as materially false, represents to me. If it represents an absence, he says, it is true; and if it represents a positive entity, it is not the idea of cold. *This is right*; but my only reason for calling the idea "materially false" is that, owing to the fact that it is obscure and confused, I am unable to judge whether or not what it represents to me is something positive which exists outside of my sensation. And hence I may be led to judge that it is something positive though in fact it may merely be an absence. (CSM II 164; AT VII 234, emphasis added)

In the above passage, Descartes acknowledges Arnauld's objection and, as a result, he clarifies that sensory ideas misrepresent their objects

[22] As I already anticipated in the Overview, it is possible to avoid this question altogether by denying that Cartesian sensations are representational. But I will argue against this reading of Cartesian sensations in Chapter 2 below.

insofar as they exhibit an obscure and confused presentation of the object of thought. Sensory ideas are ideas whose representational content is so obscure and confused that we cannot detect from immediate inspection of their presentational content what object they represent exactly.[23] Notice that although this understanding of sensory misrepresentation may still be interpreted as implying that sensory ideas refer to one object but present a different one to us (as we shall see in Chapter 3), it does not necessarily imply this interpretation. Descartes could be saying that sensory ideas misrepresent because *they present their correct objects obscurely* (that is, as having some properties that they do not actually have). This claim is consistent with DA. Sensory ideas exhibit, so to speak, a distorted image of the (correct) object of thought. And insofar as sensory ideas exhibit this confused presentational content they provide the subject matter for error. For, on the basis of their confused representation of the corporeal world, they can lead me to make the erroneous judgments, for example, that the bread I am eating is sweet or that the couch I am sitting on is white.

Having established that it is at least possible for Descartes to admit of a notion of misrepresentation that is consistent with DA, I want to address the following question next: what is the evidence that the objects of sensory ideas are bodies or properties thereof? If materially false ideas are ideas that represent obscurely and confusedly they still represent something and the object represented cannot be totally unknown to the subject.[24] But what is this object? The nature of this object can be inferred by various passages in the *Meditations.* First, in Meditation Three, Descartes includes perceptions of light and color among ideas of corporeal things (*Quantum autem ad ideas rerum corporalium*) (CSM II 29; AT VII 43). And earlier on in Meditation Three, Descartes had drawn a parallelism between hearing a noise and seeing the sun and classified both kinds of perceptions as adventitious ideas that lead us to judge that they come from things existing outside of us (CSM II 26;

[23] The association between material falsity and obscure and confused ideas was already present in Meditation Three where Descartes writes that the ideas of light and colors are obscure and confused "to the extent that I do not even know whether they are true or false, that is, whether the ideas I have of them are ideas of real things or of non-things" (CSM II 30; AT VII 43).

[24] For a similar point see Vinci (1998), p. 197 and Bolton (1986), p. 395.

AT VII 38).[25] Second, in his replies to Arnauld, Descartes writes that the idea of cold is materially false because "owing to the fact that it is obscure and confused, I am unable to judge whether or not what represents to me is something positive which exists outside our sensation" (CSM II 164; AT VII 234). This indicates that the object of the obscure idea is taken to be an object that exists outside the mind.[26] Third, the argument for the existence of material things in Meditation Six *presupposes* that all ideas of sense are ideas that exhibit bodies to the mind. It is precisely this feature of sensory perceptions that leads us to believe that they come from bodies and it is this belief that God's veracity is supposed to guarantee. Finally, and more generally, the fact that sensations represent bodies (even if not accurately) is what allows the mind–body union (of which sensations are modes) to move around successfully in the surrounding environment.[27]

In conclusion, we ought to take Descartes' definition of sensory ideas as materially false to mean, metaphorically, that sensory ideas represent bodies as other than they actually are. This happens because sensory ideas present bodies confusedly, that is, as possessing some properties that they do not actually possess. More precisely, these ideas are obscure and confused as long as they represent their correct object (i.e., a body) as if it resembled the felt sensation of redness or sweetness. Accordingly, they can lead to erroneous judgments. For example, suppose the idea of *n* represents *n* as having the properties P, F and Φ – where P stands for the property of extension, F for the property of size and Φ for the

[25] One could object that the adventitious character of hearing a noise is not sufficient to make the sensation representational. For adventitious ideas, one could argue, are complex ideas of which the non-representational sensation is only one component. The text where Descartes is supposed to suggest that adventitious ideas are compound ideas is a passage from *Conversation with Burman* (CSMK 347; AT V 165). I believe this text is insufficient to substantiate this interpretation of ideas of secondary qualities. I discuss this kind of objection again in Chapters 5 and 6 below.

[26] For a similar reading see Beyssade (1992), p. 14. One may object that the passage could be interpreted as saying that sensations – as long as they are obscure – do not reveal to introspection whether their object is a mode of mind or of matter. However, in my view, the very possibility that this alternative is posed to the mind (should I, or should I not, judge that what they represent to me exists outside the mind?), suggests that sensations indicate something outside themselves. And that's sufficient to attribute representationality to them. Thanks to Thomas Vinci for pointing out this alternative reading of the text.

[27] See Meditation Six on this, especially AT VII 81–89; CSM II 56–61.

sensible property of redness (or phenomenal redness). Now suppose (as Cartesian physics requires) that *n* (being a body) instantiates properties P and F but not Φ. Arguably, the idea is still the idea of *n* although it represents *n* inaccurately, that is, as having *some* properties that *n* does not actually have. As a result, one may judge that there are *ns* in the world that instantiate properties P, F and Φ. Our judgment would be false and its formal falsity would be generated by the material falsity of the idea, that is, by the confused way in which the object of thought is presented to the mind.[28] Descartes endorses this broader and metaphorical definition of material falsity in his replies to Arnauld. There, he writes that materially false ideas are confused ideas that provide the subject-matter for error insofar as they are "referred to something other than that of which [they] are in fact [. . .] idea[s]" (CSM II 163; AT VII 233), that is, insofar as they present their objects not as they really are but as resembling the felt sensation ("Thus if cold is simply an absence, the idea of cold is not coldness itself, as it exists objectively in the intellect, but something else, which I erroneously mistake for this absence, namely a sensation which in fact has no existence outside the intellect" CSM II 163; AT VII 233).

It is *qua* obscure and confused ideas, I contend, that ideas of sense continue to be regarded as misrepresentations of corporeal reality in Descartes' subsequent works. In the *Meditations*, sensations are said to be confused and obscure ideas that belong to the mind–body union. This becomes clear in Meditation Six where Descartes claims that our nature as a combination of mind and body (CSM II 57; AT VII 82) teaches us (erroneously) that "the heat in a body is something exactly resembling the idea of heat which is in me; or that when a body is white or green, the selfsame whiteness or greenness which I perceive through my senses is present in the body; or that in a body which is bitter or sweet there is the selfsame taste which I experience, and so on" (CSM II 57; AT VII 82).

Similarly, in Principles I.48, Descartes claims that the sensations of color, sound, smell and the like "arise from the close and intimate union of our mind with our body" (CSM I 209; AT VIIIA 23; see also CSM I 279–282; AT VIIIA 315–318); and he indicates in subsequent sections

[28] I will return to this distinction between material and formal falsity in detail in Chapter 2.

(see, especially, Principles I.46 and 66–71) that the perceptions of color and the like are confused perceptions of bodies (insofar as we perceive color and pain as if they existed in either a body or in some part of our body in a way that resembles our perception of them) and, hence, lead to erroneous judgments about the external world. Moreover, in Principles IV.200, Descartes writes, like in Meditation Three, that perceptions of color and taste "are always confused, and we do not know what they really are" (CSM I 286; AT VIIIA 324); in Principles IV.198, he claims that light, color, smell etc. are "simply various dispositions in [external] objects which make them able to set up various kinds of motions in our nerves which are required to produce all the various sensations in our soul" (CSM I 285; AT VIIIA 322–323). One possibility is, then, that perceptions of color and the like represent these "various dispositions" in external objects confusedly because they represent them as resembling the felt sensation that is caused by these dispositions.

In the *Passions of the Soul*, Descartes includes perceptual sensations (i.e., sensations of color and taste) in the general definition of the passions together with bodily sensations (i.e., hunger and pain) and the emotions (i.e., anger and joy). Generally defined, the passions of the soul are perceptions that, although they are referred to the soul (CSM I 339; AT XI 349), they also "come to our soul by means of the nerves" (CSM I 336; AT XI 345) that are put in motion by external objects. That is, perceptual sensations belong to the union of mind and body. In Part I, section 28, Descartes clarifies that we can call the passions "perceptions" in so far as we mean that they are not volitions (that is, thoughts that proceed directly from our soul and depend on it alone, CSM I 335; AT XI 342) but not insofar as we mean "evident knowledge." This is so because "[. . .] the passions are to be numbered among those perceptions which the close alliance between the soul and the body renders confused and obscure" (CSM I 339; AT XI 350). But in what sense are the sensations of color and the like obscure and confused, according to the Descartes of the *Passions of the Soul*? In various passages, Descartes indicates that these sensations represent bodies. In Part I, section 17, he writes that perceptual sensations are called passions because they are received by the soul "from the things that are *represented* by them" (CSM I 335; AT XI 342, emphasis added); and in many other sections of Part I, Descartes claims that the sensations of color, cold, light and so on are received in us from external bodies.[29] It follows that Descartes is saying that sensations are representations of their causes, that is, bodies. But they are not accurate representations. For example, in section 23 of Part I, Descartes clarifies that "when we see the light of a torch and hear the sound of a bell, the sound and the light are two different actions which, simply by producing two different movements in some of our nerves, and through them in our brain, give to the soul two different sensations" (CSM I 337; AT XI 346). However, "we refer these sensations to the subjects we suppose to be their causes in such a way that we think that we see the torch itself and hear the bell" (Ibid.) whereas in actuality we have "sensory perception merely of the movements coming from these objects" (Ibid.). In the same way, when we have the perception of cold we experience cold as if it were in the object which causes it (CSM I 337; AT XI 347) whereas the object only causes the movements in our nerves that make the mind have the sensation of cold. In conclusion, even in the *Passions of the Soul*, Descartes holds the view that perceptual sensations are confused representations of bodies insofar as they lead us to make erroneous judgment regarding them.

Having laid out Descartes' views on ideas in general and his views on sensory ideas of secondary qualities in particular, we are ready to introduce the puzzle of sensory representation.

1.4 THE PUZZLE OF SENSORY REPRESENTATION

As we saw in 1.3 above, sensory ideas are such that there is a lack of complete correspondence between the way in which the object is presented to the mind and the object the idea actually refers to. That is, a sensory idea refers to an object which does not possess all the properties that it is presented to the mind as having. For example, the idea of red "refers to something to which it does not correspond" (CSM II 163; AT VI 233) because it presents a bodily configuration resembling the felt

[29] See especially CSM I 336–337; AT XI 345–346 and CSM I 339–341, sections 22–23 and 30–34; AT XI 351–354.

sensation of redness and there is nothing (according to Descartes' physics) in the corporeal world that exactly satisfies that description.

It is this feature of sensory ideas that generates the puzzle of sensory representation. As we saw in 1.3 above, Antoine Arnauld was the first to object that Descartes' account of sensory representation is "inconsistent with [Descartes'] own principles" (CSM II 145; AT VII 206), *viz.*, the "theory" of ideas outlined in Meditation Three and its related causal principle. According to Arnauld, there cannot be an idea of cold that represents it to us as a positive thing (assuming that cold is a privation) because the idea of cold, by Descartes' own definition, "is coldness itself as it exists objectively in the intellect." And so, objects Arnauld, "if cold is merely an absence, there cannot ever be a positive idea of it, and hence there cannot be an idea which is materially false" (CSM II 145; AT VII 206).

Arnauld's point is simple but of far-reaching implications. Descartes' theory of ideas (DA) rules out the very possibility of sensory misrepresentation. If (I)–(IV) of DA are true then ideas cannot misrepresent their objects. According to (II), an idea contains the identifying description of the object and so, as (IV) implies, an idea cannot represent its object *x* as other than *x* is (on pain of not being the idea of *x*). And so, Arnauld concludes, there cannot be an idea of cold that represents cold as something positive (i.e., as a property of body resembling the felt sensation) if cold is a privation (i.e., if there is no such property of body). Arnauld continues:

> Lastly, what does the idea of cold, which you say is materially false, represent to your mind? An absence? But in that case it is true. A positive entity? But in that case it is not the idea of cold. (CSM II 146; AT VII 207)

Arnauld asks us to suppose that we learn that cold, which we have always thought to be a positive property, is a privation. Then, he continues, according to Descartes' DA, the idea of cold presents it to the mind as either the absence of heat, and in that case the idea is true, or as a positive entity, and in that case the idea is not the idea of cold. Consequently, under DA, it is impossible to have ideas that misrepresent their objects.

Incidentally, notice the similarities between Arnauld's objection and Kripke's point that a description theory cannot account for cases in which "the speaker has erroneous beliefs about some person."[30] Suppose we learn that Schmidt (rather than Gödel) proved the incompleteness of arithmetic. If the description theory were true, Kripke argues, "Gödel" would refer to whomever in fact proved the incompleteness of arithmetic, i.e., Schmidt; and, hence, when we think of Gödel as the person who proves the incompleteness theorem we would have a correct belief about a different person rather than an erroneous belief about Gödel. Similarly, as Arnauld's criticism shows, if DA were true we could not have materially false ideas, i.e., we could never have representations of the object of the idea; assuming that cold is a privation, the idea of cold as something positive would simply be the (correct) idea of a different object.

Now, as we anticipated in 1.3 above, Descartes' views on sensory misrepresentation can be interpreted in two different ways. Sensory ideas are misrepresentations either because they refer to an object that they do not present to the mind;[31] or because they present to the mind the (same) object they refer to but so confusedly and obscurely that they provide material for erroneous judgments. The difference between the two interpretations is the difference between saying that the idea *I* represents *n* as *m* and saying that the idea *I* represents *n* obscurely and confusedly as instantiating *some* properties that *n* does not actually instantiate.[32] In his replies to Arnauld, as we also saw in 1.3, Descartes indicates that we ought to interpret his claim that ideas of sense misrepresent their objects in the second sense above. But did Descartes succeed in answering Arnauld's concerns completely? Yes and no. *Yes*, because he admitted that there cannot be a complete lack of correspondence between the presentational and referential content of the idea, that is, that we cannot have an idea referring to one thing but presenting another to the mind. But, *no*, because he never denied this claim that

[30] See Kripke (1972), pp. 83–92 and p. 106.

[31] As we shall see in Chapter 3 below, Wilson (1990) and Schmaltz (1992) and (2006) lean towards this interpretation of Descartes' view on sensory misrepresentation.

[32] As will become clear in the following chapters (especially Chapters 3 and 5), depending on how one interprets Descartes' phrase *ideas of sense represent their objects as other than they are*, one is also inclined to give different *solutions* to the puzzle of misrepresentation. For the time being, however, I am only interested in showing that no matter how we interpret Descartes' view, his claim that ideas of sense are misrepresentations remains a puzzle.

sensory ideas "refer to objects with which they do not correspond" and, hence, make us err about the nature of the external world. Let me put the same point differently. Along the lines of DA, I interpret Descartes as suggesting that sensory ideas mis*present* their true objects due to their obscurity and confusion. However, an open question still remains: how does a sensory idea manage to refer to its correct object although the object to which it refers is not evident from the sensory content of the idea? How is it possible, in light of DA, for an idea of *n* to still represent *n* while mis*presenting* it?

So, no matter how we interpret Descartes' claim that sensory ideas misrepresent the material world, Arnauld-like questions remain wide open and Descartes' answer to them remains a matter of theoretical speculation. I conclude, then, that the notion of sensory misrepresentation poses a puzzle for Descartes and his interpreters. If sensory ideas are misrepresentations of their objects, they must represent them. But, then, what theory of *representation* would account for why sensory ideas represent their objects as other than they are in normal circumstances? Did Descartes hold an internalist theory of sensory representation along the lines of DA but with sufficient qualifications to accommodate cases of misrepresentations and meet Arnauld-like objections? If so, what are these qualifications? And how can sensory ideas refer to their correct objects although these objects are not evident from the sensory content of the ideas? Or, do we have to infer that Descartes held a completely different theory of sensory representation? Did he hold an externalist theory? And if he did, what kind of externalist theory did he hold? It is this puzzle, or cluster of puzzles, that I endeavor to unravel and solve in this book.

1.5 TERMINOLOGICAL CLARIFICATIONS

While introducing Descartes' theory of ideas and the puzzle of sensory representation, I also introduced some of the terminology that I will be using throughout the book. According to Descartes, ideas are modes of awareness (their formal reality) that have representational properties (their objective being/reality). The representational properties are what I call the *representational content* of ideas; and the representational content of ideas divides into two different types, *referential and presentational* content. Let me clarify these terms in turn:

Referential Content: ideas are about, or stand for, objects other than themselves (whether or not these objects actually exist).[33]

But there is more to ideas than just their objects since these objects are *presented in certain ways* and there can be different ways of presenting the same object. I call the way in which the object of the idea is presented to the mind the *presentational content* of ideas:

Presentational Content: It consists in the way in which the object of thought is cognitively presented to the mind.

But, as we saw in sections 1.2 and 1.3 above, there are at least two different types of presentational content, according to Descartes, and they amount to two very different ways in which the object of thought is cognitively accessed by the mind:

Sensory presentational content: in the case of sensory ideas, the object of thought is presented in an obscure and confused way, that is, as having some properties that it does not actually have.

Intelligible presentational content: in the case of intellectual ideas, the object of thought is presented in a clear and distinct way, that is, as having (all and only) the properties that it actually has.

Notice that the above explanation of the representational content of ideas is neutral between internalist and externalist readings. It only says that the representational content of ideas consists in their property of exhibiting an object to the mind in certain ways regardless of how this property is determined. In the following chapters, I will address the question of whether this property of *sensory* ideas is to be explained internally (along the lines of Descartes' DA) or externally (along the lines of causal or teleological theories of content). Needless to say, depending on how this question is answered the relation between the presentational and referential content of sensory ideas will also vary.

[33] I am not considering here the case of ideas of reflection, or ideas by which we may think of our own mental states.

1.6 CAVEATS

One may remark that my presentation of the puzzle of representation already betrays my stand on some basic (but not uncontroversial) exegetical issues. So, in order to dispel the initial suspicion of uncritical biases and in anticipation of the possible objection that I am begging the question with some of my opponents from the start, I will be explicit about my stand on these basic issues, briefly indicate why and refer the reader to various parts of the book where I defend my views in more detail.

I claimed above that Cartesian sensations are (a) intrinsically representational;[34] (b) they represent (or seem to represent) external objects; and that (c) they *mis*represent external objects. However, (a)–(c) have all been questioned in the literature. Many Descartes scholars would deny (a) because they interpret Descartes as drawing a wedge between sensations and truly representative ideas. According to this reading, Cartesian sensations are *qualia* and as such they are intrinsically non-representational mental states. I will argue extensively against this reading in Chapters 2 and 5. But let me just point out here that the very passage in Meditation Three where Descartes introduces the notion of material falsity (discussed in 1.3 above) seems to provide strong evidence against this interpretation (insofar as Descartes claims there that sensory ideas represent "non-things *as things*"). Besides, Descartes calls ideas of sense "images" and this suggests that they are representational.

Most of the scholars who agree with (a) above also agree with (b), that is, with the claim that Cartesian sensations represent bodies or properties thereof (although confusedly). But some scholars have criticized this reading and maintain instead that, according to Descartes, ideas of sense represent modes of the mind (or *qualia*). Nelson (1996), for example, has argued that ideas of secondary qualities are intrinsically representational but that they intrinsically represent modes of the mind. His view is that ideas of secondary qualities are clearly and distinctly understood as ideas of *qualia* (or modes of the mind) and as such they

[34] As will become clear in Chapter 2, when I say that Cartesian sensations are intrinsically representational, I mean that they exhibit intentionality inherently or prior to any judgment.

reality-represent modes of the mind.[35] I will defend (b) against this alternative reading in Chapter 2 and throughout the book.[36] Suffice it to say here that I believe that this reading is both textually unsupported and theoretically unsound. Descartes always discusses ideas of secondary qualities in the context of his discussion of ideas of material things and the very proof of the existence of material things in Meditation Six assumes that ideas of sense are ideas of bodies.[37] Besides, the attribution to Descartes of the view that the mind "represents" its sensations to itself is very unCartesian. Ideas are the ways by which objects become cognitively accessible to the mind. But sensations do not need to become cognitively accessible to us by way of ideas. They can certainly be made the object of our attention by reflecting on them but this hardly implies that this is the way they are normally experienced by us. The idea of red, for example, is not the idea that presents the sensation of redness to me; rather *it is* the sensation *of something red*.

Finally, it is possible to challenge the pivotal assumption of the present book, that is, that Descartes held the view that ideas of secondary qualities are misrepresentations. Alison Simmons, for example, argues that Descartes holds a teleological account of the representationality of sensation, according to which sensations represent what they do in virtue of their biological function.[38] Since the mind-union, in order to navigate the environment successfully, needs to know which bodies sensations represent, sensations represent bodies. And insofar as sensations represent bodies successfully, Simmons concludes, they are "materially true." It is only the mistaken assumption that, according to Descartes, resemblance is a necessary condition for representation that leads to the (also mistaken) conclusion that Cartesian sensations are misrepresentations.

I will discuss Simmons' views, and teleological accounts in general, in Chapter 4. But let me say the following now. I agree with Simmons that, according to Descartes, resemblance is not a necessary condition for representation. Descartes held a correspondence theory of truth and a satisfaction theory of reference and neither notion has anything to do

35 See Nelson (1996), p. 23.

36 A brief discussion of Nelson's views is to be found in Chapter 2.

37 See, for example, CSM II 29; AT VII 43 and CSM II 54–55; AT VII 78–79.

38 See Simmons (1999).

with resemblance.[39] But we should keep in mind that Descartes defines truth as a matter of correspondence between the clear and distinct ideas of the intellect and reality. And as long as ideas of sense are obscure and confused (as opposed to clear and distinct) they are misrepresentations of reality. They are not misrepresentations of reality because they fail to resemble physical reality. Rather, they are misrepresentations of reality because the object presented to the mind (for example, a property of body resembling the sensation of red) falls short of the clear and distinct *representation* of physical reality (and, hence, fails to correspond to the true object of thought which is determined by the clear and distinct ideas of the intellect).[40] Besides, the fact that sensations are misrepresentations of their objects does not imply that they fail to carry "some truth." As long as they represent something in the outside world they are partly veridical. But this conclusion is not enough to make sensory ideas "materially true" and in fact Descartes never calls them "materially true."[41]

In conclusion, although I inevitably took a stand on some basic interpretative matters in setting up the exegetical problem under discussion, I will argue for my views and defend them against others in the course of the book.

[39] For a reading of Descartes' conception of truth as consistency of belief see Frankfurt (1970). I cannot embark on a full discussion of Frankfurt's views here. I will just say that I disagree with this reading on textual grounds. Descartes indicates in many places that he holds a correspondence theory of truth. See, for example, Letter to Mersenne, 16 October 1639, CSMK 139; AT II 597.

[40] That is, given that truth is related to clarity and distinctness, sensory ideas are "false" insofar as they fall short of clarity and distinctness.

[41] For an implicit criticism of Simmons' (1999) contention that Cartesian sensations are materially true along similar lines, see Brown (2006), p. 109.

2

Non-Representationalist Solutions: Cartesian Sensations as *Qualia*

According to a widespread interpretation, Cartesian sensations are devoid of the property of representationality. They are instead (what in the contemporary literature are called) *qualia* insofar as they present themselves as non-relational or purely qualitative features of experience.[1] On this interpretation, Descartes' view would be that in perceiving colors one is merely experiencing the subjective feel of redness or blueness rather than perceiving external bodies as red or blue.

Nicholas Malebranche interpreted Cartesian sensations this way. According to Malebranche, Descartes held the view that sensations of color, taste, pain and the like "are nothing but modes of the mind" (S I.i.2) because they neither represent nor seem to represent anything in the external world (S I.x.48; see also S I.vii).[2] Since then many scholars have followed in Malebranche's footsteps in interpreting Descartes this way.[3]

[1] Notoriously, the very definition of *qualia* is controversial. On this see Block (1994) and (2003). In this context, I am concerned only with the question of whether Cartesian sensations are *qualia* in the sense that they lack representational content. This is the question which has concerned Descartes scholars. And this is the way Loar (2003), Tye (2002) and Crane (2001), for example, address the problem of *qualia* in the contemporary debate.

[2] On this see Nadler (1992), chapter two. Watson (1966) argues that the view that Cartesian sensations aren't representational was held by many later Cartesians. See especially, Watson (1966), chapters three and five.

[3] See, for example, Alanen (1994) and (2003); Field (1993); MacKenzie (1990); Nelson (1996); Vinci (1998); Wilson (1978). The attribution of this interpretation of Descartes to Alanen and Nelson needs qualification since it may not appear immediately obvious that they hold it. I attribute this view to Alanen on the basis of the following claims: "[m]aterial falsity [...] occurs in the ideas not of the second but of the third level of sensory perception, which involves unnoticed or unconscious judgments" (Alanen (1994), p. 244); and "[...] material falsity would differ from formal falsity not because

Moreover, this interpretation of Cartesian sensations as *qualia* is seen by contemporary philosophers of mind as part and parcel of Descartes' internalist account of mental content (i.e., the view that mental states are individuated non-relationally) and its (allegedly) related skepticism of the veil of ideas.[4] It is Descartes, after all, who opened up the problem of our knowledge of an external world and created an epistemological gap between the mind and the world. And Cartesian *qualia* are perfect candidates for those third entities between the mind and the world. For example, one may argue that Descartes' dream and deceiver arguments are arguments for *qualia* as follows. Suppose Mary is dreaming of a red rose. What Mary is dreaming of is not a real red rose because Mary isn't seeing anything. So, the color Mary is experiencing is a property of her own experience. But if dreaming is indistinguishable from veridical experience, then *qualia* occur in veridical experience also.[5]

no judgments are involved, but because the judgments involved are implicit and unnoticed, and therefore difficult to distinguish from the actual sensations, giving us thus material for error" (Ibid., p. 246). And I attribute this interpretation to Nelson, as we shall see presently, because he denies that Cartesian sensations represent anything external. Richard Field, as we shall see below, distinguishes between ideas of sense and sensations and he takes the latter – qua *qualia* – to be the objects of the former. Thomas Vinci agrees with Margaret Wilson that, in the *Principles* (especially *Principles* I.71 and I.46), Descartes came to think of sensations of color and the like as non-representational states because colors and the like are modes of the mind. See Vinci (1998) chapter seven (especially 7.9) and Wilson (1978), chapter three (especially pp. 118–119).

[4] This is suggested, for example, by Loar (2003). In Dennett (1988), Dennett summarizes the traditional view of *qualia* as attributing to them the following features: ineffability, intrinsicality, privacy and direct accessibility. It's not hard to see how this tradition can be traced back to Descartes. See Dennett (1988), p. 229.

[5] For this kind of example, see Tye (2002), p. 447. Notice that the interpretation of Descartes as holding a representationalist theory of the mind according to which ideas are "third entities" that mediate our knowledge of the world goes back to Thomas Reid and is accepted by Richard Rorty and Jonathan Bennett (among many others). On this see Yolton (1984), pp. 3–41 (although Yolton himself wishes to overthrow this interpretation of Descartes). I do not mean to suggest that Descartes didn't hold a representational theory of mind. But holding a representational theory of mind doesn't necessarily mean reifying mental states and reifying mental states doesn't necessarily imply robbing them of intentionality. More generally, there is an inclination to burden Descartes with the introduction of *qualia* simply because, according to Descartes, it is (conceivably) possible to have sensations without there being an external world that causes these sensations in us. But notice that the fact that this is a possible scenario for Descartes doesn't even begin to support the view that sensations present themselves as purely qualitative features of experience. The deceiver and dream arguments of Meditation One are perfectly compatible with sensations *seeming* to represent an external world.

Finally, this reading of Cartesian sensations fits the more general view that the Rationalist Descartes denied that the senses play any cognitive role in the search for truth. This role is allotted to the intellect alone. Sensations are mere impressionistic modes of the mind and do not serve any cognitive purpose.[6]

If this non-representationalist interpretation of Cartesian sensations were correct, the puzzle of sensory representation would be a red herring. However, we cannot dismiss the puzzle so easily since the non-representationalist interpretation of Cartesian sensations is *not* correct. This chapter defends this claim. First, I will establish that the arguments and textual evidence offered in support of the non-representationalist interpretation fail to prove that Cartesian sensations are *qualia* (2.2–2.4). Second, I will argue that there are textual and theoretical reasons for believing exactly the opposite, that is, that Descartes held that sensations are intrinsically intentional (2.5–2.6).

2.1 THE ARGUMENTS IN SUPPORT OF THE NON-REPRESENTATIONALIST INTERPRETATION

Malebranche distinguished between sensations and ideas.[7] According to Malebranche, in the case of sensations of color, taste and the like we must keep separate the sensation proper (i.e., the what-it-feels-like-to-see-red, for example) from the natural judgment of projecting what the mind senses onto external bodies (see S I.x.52–53).[8] Sensations of color and the like are devoid of intrinsic intentionality. The fact that when we feel pain or see color we see them in objects, explains Malebranche, is only the result of an involuntary natural judgment (S I.x.52–53 and

[6] See for example MacKenzie (1990), p. 125: "For Descartes sensations are inherently non-veridical and can play no role in the mind's search after truth."

[7] Despite the fact that Malebranche uses "idea" in general to signify anything that is immediately perceived by the mind he wants to distinguish ideas in the strictest sense from sensations proper (see S I.i and S Elucidation III. 561). It is in this strict sense that I use the terms "idea" and "sensation" here.

[8] The same distinction between sensation proper and an act of judgment doesn't seem to apply to the case of sensation of extension, according to Malebranche. See S I.vii.

S I.xiii.68–69). The intentionality of sensations is then inherited from a judgment as opposed to being intrinsic to the sensation. On the contrary, on Malebranche's view, ideas have intrinsic representational content because they represent objects in the external world and their properties. Our idea of extension, for example, suffices to provide information about all the properties of bodies (S III.vii.237 and S Elucidation III. 561).

Malebranche's view on sensations of secondary qualities is supposed to be Descartes' legacy. As Simmons puts it, the interpretation of sensations as *qualia* is believed to be Descartes' legacy because "having excised colors, sounds [. . .] from the corporeal world [. . .] [Descartes] relocated them in the mind in the form of sensations that do little more than give an ornamental [. . .] flair to our sense perceptual experience."[9] The argument by which Malebranche attributes this view to Descartes is precisely along these lines:

(1) According to Cartesian physics, bodies are modes of *res extensa, viz.*, modifications of the essential property of body (i.e., extension).
(2) Therefore, colors, tastes, pains and the like are banished from the corporeal world.
(3) Therefore, according to Descartes, sensations of pain, color and the like do not resemble any real quality of corporeal substance.
(4) Therefore, Cartesian sensations are devoid of any intrinsic representational content. They are mere modes of the mind.
(5) Therefore, any appearance of representational content that sensations exhibit must be *inherited* from the implicit judgment we make that what is present to the mind has a similar counterpart in reality.[10]

Some contemporary scholars have attributed to Descartes the view that sensations of color and the like are *qualia* on the basis of similar arguments. I will briefly present two different variations of Malebranche's original argument in the following two sub-sections.

[9] See Simmons (1999), p. 347.
[10] See S I.i; x; xiii. On this see Nadler (1989), chapter three and Nadler (1992), chapter two. Simmons (1999), pp. 347–349, also attributes this argument to Malebranche.

2.1.1 Wilson's Argument

Margaret Wilson argues that Descartes, in *Principles* I.66–71, distinguishes sensations from other perceptions as follows.[11] Since sensations of color do not resemble any real property in things (CSM I 216–218; AT VIIIA 32–34) and, so, they "do not represent anything located outside our thought" (CSM I 219; AT VIIIA 35), colors and tastes are exhibited to the mind *as* sensations (CSM I 219; AT VIIIA 35). On the contrary, since our clear and distinct perception of size, shape and so forth "exactly corresponds" to real properties of objects (CSM I 218; AT VIIIA 34) size and shape are exhibited to the mind *as of* things (CSM I 219; AT VIIIA 35).[12]

However, Wilson continues, Descartes points out that we don't notice the difference between these two kinds of perceptions. When we perceive colors in objects, writes Descartes, "we cannot find any resemblance between the colour [. . .] and that which we experience in our sensation. But this is something we do not take account of; and what is more there are many other features such as size, shape and number which we clearly perceive to be actually or at least possibly in objects in a way exactly corresponding to our sensory perception and understanding" (CSM I 218; AT VIIIA 34). Because we neglect the difference between perceptions of color and perceptions of size, we erroneously assimilate the two kinds of perceptions and, so, we make the mistake of "judging that what is called colour in objects is something exactly like the colour of which we have sensory awareness" (CSM I 218; AT VIIIA 35).

[11] Wilson (1978), pp. 118–119. As I already noted in the Overview, according to Wilson (1978), Descartes changed his views on sensations over the years. In the *Meditations*, he would still hold that sensations are representational.

[12] Notice that it is unclear (both in Wilson and in Descartes) whether the distinction is between the sensory perceptions of primary and secondary qualities or between the sensory perceptions of secondary qualities and the clear understanding of primary qualities. The issue is complicated since it is not clear in what sense the sensory perception of size "exactly corresponds to" the primary qualities of things. Since it is at least unproblematic that, according to Descartes, the clear and distinct understanding of these features exactly corresponds to real properties, I assumed that the above distinction is between the clear and distinct understanding of primary qualities and the sensory perception of secondary qualities.

Notice that, as in Malebranche's argument, Wilson argues that (i) sensations proper aren't representational because they do not resemble any real property of bodies; and that (ii) the representational content of Cartesian sensations is the result of a judgment that in turn is the result of confusing sensations with ideas.[13]

2.1.2 MacKenzie's Argument

Ann Wilbur MacKenzie agrees with Margaret Wilson that Descartes distinguishes between mere sensations and representative perceptions of extension and figure. She also agrees with Wilson that what causes the error of believing that colors exist in bodies is not the intrinsic intentionality of sensations but the fact that mere sensations are mistakenly associated with the really representative perception of extension, figure, and size. She argues for the lack of intrinsic intentionality of sensations as follows:

(1) There is an *ontological* difference between secondary and primary qualities. The former are qualities of embodied minds, *viz.*, they are "qualia which embodied minds 'have.'"[14] The latter are real qualities of bodies.

(2) "Descartes' [views about] the ontological status of [secondary qualities] puts pressure on his view that human sensing is in general a kind of representing."[15]

(3) Therefore, Descartes distinguishes two different categories of sensory perception: (i) in sensing secondary qualities we are having mere sensations devoid of any representational content; (ii) in sensing primary qualities we are acquainted with real properties of things.[16]

[13] See Wilson (1978), p. 119: "[According to Descartes, our inclination to believe that colors exist outside the mind does not] result from an intrinsic feature of sensations [...]. Rather, it is supposed to result from their confusing *association* with the really representative perceptions of extension, figure and motion."

[14] MacKenzie (1990), p. 114.

[15] Ibid., p. 115.

[16] See Mackenzie (1990), p. 115: "My suggestion here is that Descartes' work on sense in humans fragments, as a result of Descartes' concerns about the ontological status of [secondary qualities]." Descartes' considered view, according to MacKenzie, is that colors are basic properties of the mind rather than being non-basic properties of bodies. See MacKenzie (1990), pp. 114–116 and pp. 122–124.

Again, the key feature of Malebranche's archetypical argument is in place here. The sensation of red, for example, does not represent the property of being red because there is no property of being red in objects that resembles the felt sensation. The *sensation* of red is an instance of the property of being red. Consequently, sensations proper aren't representational.

In conclusion, the non-representationalist interpretation of Cartesian sensations consists of two related theses: (1) Cartesian sensations are the purely qualitative aspect of conscious experience. That is, they are *qualia* devoid of any intrinsic intentionality; and (2) the intentionality they "appear" to exhibit is only the result of an implicit (and illicit) judgment.

As we saw above, what motivates this interpretation is a cluster of diverse arguments with a common-core. However, as I will argue in section 2.2, there are several reasons to doubt the conclusiveness of the above argument(s).

2.2 PROBLEMS WITH THE CORE-ARGUMENT FOR THE NON-REPRESENTATIONALIST INTERPRETATION

The core-argument for the non-representationalist interpretation embodies the following key inference:

(KI): There are no real properties of bodies that *resemble* the sensation of color and the like, according to Cartesian physics; therefore, sensations of color and the like do not *represent* anything outside the mind.

However, this inference is problematic. Firstly, notice that (KI) assumes that *resemblance*, according to Descartes, is a necessary condition for representation. However, this seems to be the wrong assumption to make in light of Descartes' explicit claim that sensations represent their objects *as other than* they are (CSM II 30; AT VII 44; and CSM II 163–164 and AT VII 233–235). And, in fact, alternative accounts of the representationality of Cartesian sensations have been offered in the literature. It has been argued that although sensations fail to resemble real properties of bodies they may still represent these properties either in virtue of a causal connection with the environment (Schmaltz (1992) and Wilson (1990)) or in virtue of the biological function of sensations (Simmons (1999)) or in virtue of a latent intellectual content (see Bolton (1986)). All these alternative explanations will be discussed in the ensuing chapters.

Secondly, (and relatedly) (KI) is invalid in light of the distinction Descartes draws between clear and distinct ideas, on the one hand, and obscure and confused ideas on the other. According to Descartes, the clear and distinct ideas of the intellect delimit the boundaries of what's real. The notion of reality relates to the notion of clear and distinct perception, at least in this sense: only with clear and distinct ideas are we without doubt about the object being represented, its reality and degree thereof. However, according to Descartes, there is a class of ideas – i.e., "materially false ideas" – that fall short of clarity and distinctness. They appear to represent something ("since there can be no ideas which are not as it were of things" CSM II 30; AT VII 44) although they "contain so little clarity and distinctness that they do not enable [us] to tell" (Ibid.) what the nature of the object being represented is or whether it is real at all. So, ideas of secondary qualities are representational (i.e., they appear to represent something) although their representational content is so obscure that we cannot tell from analyzing them whether they represent something real (see CSM II 30; AT VII 44; CSM II 164; AT VII 234) let alone *what* the real objects of the ideas are. Suppose, for example, that an object *x* with degree of reality R1 is contained objectively in the idea. In the case of obscure and confused ideas, this object is contained in the idea but the obscurity of the way in which it is presented by the senses veils its exact degree of reality (and this may lead us to doubt whether the idea is representing anything real at all). (KI) assumes that a lack of objective reality ("There are no real properties of bodies that *resemble* the sensation of color") is sufficient to establish a lack of representationality ("therefore, sensations of color [. . .] do not *represent* anything outside the mind"). But even if we acknowledge that sensory ideas fail to exhibit objective reality *on their sleeves* because there is no real property of bodies that *resembles* the felt color sensation, it does not follow that these ideas fail to represent altogether. On the contrary, Descartes claims that sensory ideas represent colors *as if they were real* properties of bodies. Undoubtedly this is obscure and confused representation, and Descartes never denies it. It still remains unexplained why color sensations represent colors *as if* they were real properties of bodies even though there are no real properties of bodies that resemble the sensations. But this is a different issue and it could be answered in a number of different ways, as we shall see in the following chapters. Suffice it to say here that one possibility is that sensory ideas lack objective reality *only* insofar as they fall short of clear and distinct perception. But the fact that they fail to exhibit objective reality *on their sleeves* (because they are obscure and confused ideas) does not rule out that they possess objective reality. Their objective reality may not be evident to us as long as we are immersed in the sensory apprehension of the corporeal world or until the intellect has examined the confused sensory content. And, so, although sensory ideas appear not to have any objective reality because there is nothing in the corporeal world that *resembles* color sensations, they may still represent something real in the corporeal world (and, hence, exhibit representationality) in virtue of "containing" an objective reality that is not (yet) evident to the *sensing* subject.[17] The real issue consists in establishing what determines this objective reality and this issue will be abundantly addressed below.

One may attempt to salvage (KI) from the above criticisms by rephrasing it as follows:

(KI)[1]: The sensation of red cannot represent a property of bodies because the sensation of red is an instance of the property of being red.[18]

Certainly this is a possible way of reading (KI). But even assuming that this rephrasing captures Descartes' views on the nature of secondary qualities – and I have my doubts, as will become clear below – this rephrasing does not

[17] Some commentators have suggested that Cartesian sensations exhibit "representative character" in so far as they exhibit various things to us but lack objective reality. Their argument is as follows. Descartes needs to attribute representative character to sensory ideas in order to explain why we make erroneous judgments about the nature of physical reality; however, Descartes also holds that sensations lack objective reality because they are caused by nothing ("if [these ideas] are false, that is, represent non-things, I know by the natural light that they arise from nothing" CSM II 30; AT VII 44) and represent non-things ("I think of [colors, taste and the like] only in a very obscure and confused way, to the extent that I do not even know whether they are true or false" CSM II 30; AT VII 43); so, the notion of representative character is independent of the notion of objective reality. See Wilson (1978), pp. 100–114. For a similar view see Normore (1986), pp. 225–230. I disagree that Descartes' attribution of representationality to sensations is independent of his attributing objective reality to them. In fact, in both Wilson (1978) and Normore (1986) the notion of representative character remains unexplained. What Cartesian doctrine would explain this (primitive?) property of sensations? The lack of an answer may, in the end, be not so surprising. Descartes' theory of representation consists in his theory of objective being and reality and, so, it is no surprise that if we separate the notions of objective reality from that of representation we are left with no explanation of the latter.

[18] The difference between (KI)[1] and (KI) is that the latter only says that there are no properties of body that resemble sensations of color and the like but it doesn't take a stand on the ontological status of secondary properties. (KI)[1] clearly does.

rescue (KI) from the above criticism. All that can be inferred from the claim that the sensation of red is an instance of the property of being red is that the sensation of red *ought not* to represent redness as a property of bodies. But from the fact that "it ought not to" it does not follow that "it does not."

Moreover, (KI)[1] makes clear that the inference for the non-representationalist interpretation moves from an ontological claim about the nature of secondary qualities (according to which secondary qualities would be modes of the mind) to a claim about that property of the mind that is called "intentionality." But how can we infer from this ontological claim about the nature of secondary qualities anything about the intentionality of the mind? What exactly is the argument that if colors are modes of the mind then the mind does not present colors *as if* they were properties of bodies? Maybe there is a relation between these two claims, but I don't see any explicit explanation of this relation and we are in desperate need of one if the case for Cartesian *qualia* is to be made. In the absence of such explanation, the claim that the sensation of red is an instance of the property of being red is, at best, just begging the question against supporters of a representational reading of sensations.

Finally, it is not obvious that Descartes had set views on the ontological status of secondary qualities. (KI)[1] takes for granted that, according to Descartes, secondary qualities are nothing but *qualia* that embodied minds have. However, I am inclined to believe that Descartes' views on the matter were more complicated than this. Consider the following passages from the *Principles*:

> [...] the properties *in* external objects to which we apply the terms light, colour, smell, taste, sound, heat and cold [...] are [...] simply various dispositions in those objects which make them able to set up various kinds of motions in our nerves which are required to produce all the various sensations in our soul. (CSM I 285; AT VIIIA 323, emphasis added)

> [light, colors and so on] are nothing else *in* the objects [...] but certain dispositions depending on size, shape and motions [of their parts]. (CSM I 285; AT VIIIA 323, emphasis added. See also CSM I 217; AT VIIIA 33)

These passages suggest that colors and the like are indeed properties *in* objects that do not resemble the felt color sensations although they play a causal role in our having color sensations. Notice that this is compatible with attributing to Descartes a view that he certainly held, that is, the view that there is something qualitative in consciousness when we experience colors and the like. The above passages provide evidence that, according to Descartes, sensations of color and the like do represent some real property of bodies although they misrepresent it as resembling the felt-sensation. So, for example, although the sensation of red has a qualitative aspect, it still represents (in virtue of a relation other than resemblance) a yet unknown bodily state (i.e., some configuration of the size and shape of the particles that make up matter) that is the cause of the sensation.[19]

For all of the above reasons, I find the core-argument for the non-representationalist interpretation inconclusive. But even assuming that a supporter of this interpretation may acknowledge the problems raised above, she may insist that there is independent textual evidence for her interpretation. In the following section, I will examine this textual evidence and argue that it does not provide incontrovertible support for reading Cartesian sensations as non-representational mental states.

2.3 THE TEXTUAL EVIDENCE FOR THE NON-REPRESENTATIONALIST INTERPRETATION

In Principles I.66 and I.68, Descartes writes that sensations, understood clearly and distinctly, are nothing but *modes of awareness*:

> [Sensations] may be clearly perceived provided that we take great care in our judgments concerning them to include no more than what is strictly contained in our perception – no more than that of which we have *inner awareness.* (CSM I 216; AT VIIIA 32, emphasis added)

> In order to distinguish what is *clear* [. . .] from what is *obscure,* we must be very careful to note that pain and colour and so on are clearly and distinctly perceived when they are regarded merely as *sensations* or *thoughts.* (CSM I 217; AT VIIIA 33, emphasis added)

[19] For a similar view see Sellars (1978). Thanks to Bryson Brown for referring me to this article. One could read the above passages as expressing the mistaken judgment about colors made by the vulgar as opposed to expressing Descartes' own considered view. However, there is no indication, in the text, that this is the case.

These passages are taken to offer conclusive evidence that Descartes holds that sensations are *qualia.* Notice, however, that the contrast being drawn here is between the obscure and confused, and the clear and distinct perceptions of sensible qualities. But drawing this distinction is compatible with maintaining that the obscure and confused perception of color presents color *as* a property of things (rather than as a mere sensation). And it should come as no surprise that Descartes claims that sensations clearly understood are modes of awareness. It is a basic tenet of Descartes' epistemology and metaphysics that the content of sense experience can be amended by attending to the clear and distinct ideas of the intellect. Once we have reinterpreted the confused content of experience according to the ideas of the intellect we can see that the true object of, for example, the idea of red is a particular arrangement of the insensible geometrical and mechanical properties of matter and, hence, that there is nothing in corporeal reality that resembles the felt sensation of red. So, Descartes' claim in Principles I.66 and I.68 that colors, *clearly* understood, are only modes of awareness is still compatible with his maintaining that the obscure and confused ideas of color presents color *as* a property of bodies. In fact, it seems precisely this representational feature of ideas of color that explains why we make the rush judgment that in seeing colors we are seeing "a thing located outside us which closely resembled the idea of color that we experienced within us" (CSM I 216; AT VIIIA 32).

Another passage often cited as providing incontrovertible support for the non-representationalist interpretation is from Principles I.71:

> [...] sensations of tastes, smells, sounds, heat, cold, light, colours and so on [...] *do not represent anything located outside our thought.* At the same time the mind perceived sizes, shapes, motions and so on, which were presented to it *not as sensations, but as things,* or modes of things, existing (or at least capable of existing) outside thought, *although it was not yet aware of the difference between things and sensations.* (CSM I 219; AT VIIIA 35, emphasis added)

In this passage, Descartes, according to the supporters of the non-representationalist interpretation, claims that (a) sensations lack representational content altogether; and (b) colors unlike size and shape, are exhibited to the mind *as* sensations rather than *as* things. But notice that when Descartes writes that sensations of color and the like "do not represent anything located outside our thought" he may simply be repeating that these sensations do not represent anything real located outside of us *that resembles the felt sensation.* In fact, Descartes claims that sensations represent real properties of things located outside of us in the section of the *Principles* immediately preceding the one in the quoted passage. In Principles I.70, he writes that "when we say that we perceive colours in objects, this is really just the same as saying that we perceive *something in the objects whose nature we do not know*, but which produces in us a certain very clear and vivid sensation which we call the sensation of colour" (CSM I 218; AT VIIIA 34). *Contra* (a) above then, a sensation of color, according to Descartes, does represent a real property of bodies (i.e., a mode of *res extensa* that produces the sensation in us) *without* resembling it. We simply do not know this until the intellect has examined the matter. As to claim (b) above, notice that Descartes is saying, in the passage quoted from Principles I.71, that although we ought to draw a distinction between properties such as colors and sizes (so that the former are presented "as sensations" and the latter "as things"), the mind *initially* is not aware of this distinction. That is, Descartes acknowledges that the mind presents *both* kinds of sensations *as if of things.*

Finally, there is the passage from Descartes' Sixth Set of Replies where he distinguishes three grades of sensation. The first grade of sensation, according to Descartes, comprises only the physiological and mechanical aspect of sensory perception. The second grade "comprises [. . .] the perceptions of pain, pleasure, thirst, hunger, colours, sound, taste, smell, heat, cold and the like" (CSM II 294; AT VII 437). And the third grade includes "the judgments about things outside of us which we have been accustomed to make from our earliest years" (CSM II 295; AT VII 437). Then, Descartes goes on to describe the second and third grades of sensation using the example of the blind man with a stick from his *Optics* (CSM I 152–175; AT VI 81–147):

> [. . .] the second grade [of sensation] [. . .] extends to the mere perception of the *colour and light* reflected from the stick [. . .]. Nothing more than this should be referred to the *sensory faculty*, if we wish to distinguish it carefully from the *intellect.* But suppose that, as *a result* of being affected by this sensation of color, I judge that a stick, located outside of me, is coloured. And suppose that on the basis of the extension of the colour and its boundaries together with its position in relation to the parts of the brain, I make a *rational* calculation (*ratiociner*) about the *size, shape and distance* of the stick: *although the reasoning*

is commonly assigned to the senses [...] *it is clear that it depends solely on the intellect (a solo intellectu).* [...] I demonstrated in the Optics how size and shape can be perceived by reasoning alone (*per solam ratiocinationem*). [The reason why we mistakenly think that we perceive size and so on through the senses alone] is that we make the calculation and judgment at great speed because of habit. (CSM II 295; AT VII 437–438, emphasis added)

The above description of the second and third grades of sensation (and their relation) is taken to imply that sensations *per se* aren't representational and the representational content they exhibit is only the result of an implicit judgment.[20] However, as I will show next, there is nothing in this passage that uncontroversially supports this reading. Once we read the passage in light of the *Optics* (the text Descartes explicitly refers to in the above passage) it becomes clear that the distinction that Descartes is interested in drawing here is between the perception of sensible qualities such as color and light, on the one hand, and size and shape, on the other hand. Descartes is repeating what he had argued in the *Optics*, that is, that "light and color [are] the only qualities belonging properly to the sense of sight" (CSM I 167; AT VI 130); whereas it is the intellect that, "as if by some natural geometry" (CSM I 170; AT VI 137) "sees" the distance, size and shape of bodies (CSM I 169–173; AT VI 134–143).[21] But notice that neither saying that only colors and light are (strictly speaking) *sensed* nor saying the perception of the size and shape of bodies is the result of a judgment establishes by itself that colors and light are sensed as properties of the mind. So, the possibility that the sensation of color presents color as a property of things without requiring any *reasoning* is left wide open. And so, the distinction between the perception of properties such as color (as involving the sensory faculty) and the "perception" of the size and shape of things (as involving a judgment) does not by itself establish that sensations lack intentionality unless it is already assumed that, according to Descartes, we can talk of intentionality only where a judgment is involved. But this is what we are trying to establish.

[20] See especially Alanen (1994), pp. 243–246; and Field (1993), p. 328.

[21] It is worth noticing that there is disagreement as to what exactly the role of the intellect is supposed to be in the third grade of sensation. On this see Simmons (2003), p. 555.

But even looking at the passage above independently of the *Optics* we can see that it doesn't incontrovertibly show that Descartes thought that sensations lack intrinsic intentionality. In the above passage, Descartes writes that the mere perception of color and light reflected from the stick belongs to the second grade of sensation. Then, as *a result* of "being affected by this sensation of color, I judge that a stick, located outside me, is coloured" and this judgment – Descartes writes – belongs to the third grade of sensation. The third grade of sensation is distinguished from the second because only the latter involves implicit or explicit judgment.[22] And Descartes is here saying nothing different from what he writes in many other places. For example, in Meditation Six, Descartes writes that "from the fact that I perceive by my senses a great variety of colours, sounds, smells, as well as differences in heat, hardness and the like, I am correct *in inferring* that the bodies which are the sources of these various sensory perceptions possess differences corresponding to them, though perhaps not resembling them" (CSM II 56; AT VII 81; see also CSM I 168; AT VI 133). But notice that the claim that the (implicit or explicit) judgment *is based* on the sensory perception of sensible qualities like colors does not by itself tell us anything about *how* these qualities are presented by the senses. And *if* it does suggest anything about how these qualities are perceived by the senses it suggests the opposite of what the supporters of the non-representationalist interpretation want. The very fact that Descartes writes that "as *a result* of being affected by this sensation of color, [we] judge that a stick, located outside of me, is coloured" seems to require that the sensation of color presents itself *as if* of things.[23] Besides, if the sensation of color presented color as a property of the mind rather than as a property of bodies how could we even start to infer that there are colored objects outside of me? How could any judgment result from this sensation, as Descartes suggests?

[22] For an interesting discussion of what kind of judgment may be involved in the third degree of sensation see Simmons (2003), pp. 563–569. This is a topic of considerable scholarly dispute. However, I do not need to take a stand on this issue in this context. My point is that the fact that a judgment occurs at the third grade of sensation due to the use of the intellect does not imply that sensations are perceived as non-representational at the second grade.

[23] For a similar point see Simmons (2003), p. 560.

In conclusion, a close analysis of the textual evidence that is considered indisputable evidence for the non-representationalist interpretation reveals that this evidence is not so indisputable.

2.4 VARIANTS OF THE NON-REPRESENTATIONALIST INTERPRETATION AND THEIR PROBLEMS

On the basis of this textual evidence, some scholars have maintained that since Cartesian sensations (clearly and distinctly perceived) are *qualia*, sensory ideas such as the ideas of red and cold are either intrinsic ideas of modes of the mind (Nelson (1996)) or are ideas of the intellect that represent sensations (Field (1993)). I regard these views as variants of the non-representationalist interpretation to the extent that they deny that sensations intrinsically represent bodies (either because sensations would intrinsically represent themselves or because it is the intellect that refers sensations to a physical reality). These two views, however, differ from the non-representationalist interpretation introduced in 2.1 because neither Nelson nor Field maintains that the representationality of sensation is inherited from a judgment. It is either intrinsic to the idea (Nelson (1996)) or a function of the intellect (Field (1993)).

Since these variants of the non-representationalist interpretation challenge my central claim that sensations represent corporeal reality, I want to discuss them in more detail and explain why I disagree with them.

2.4.1 Nelson's Argument

According to Nelson (1996), Descartes' view is that the ideas of red and cold are ideas of themselves, that is, they are ideas that (intrinsically) represent modes of the mind (or *qualia*). His argument is:

(1) Cartesian sensations are *ideas* of cold and red, that is, they have objective reality insofar as they are ideas *of things*;[24]

[24] Although, Nelson admits, we may not know the exact reality that is being represented insofar as these ideas are obscure and confused. See Nelson (1996), pp. 17–18.

(2) Ideas, by their objective reality, represent the degree of formal reality of its object (or cause) (according to the causal principles of Meditation Three); and "reality-representation is intrinsic to the idea."[25]

(3) In Principles I.68–71, Descartes writes that cold and the like are nothing but sensations (when clearly understood);

So, (C1), the idea of cold intrinsically represents a *quale* (or sensation);[26]

So, (C2), ideas of cold and the like are ideas of *qualia*. They are ideas that have sensations as their objects.

I want to point out several difficulties with this argument. First, premise (3) *assumes* without further argument that Descartes' considered view is that the sensation of cold is an instance of the property of being cold. But, as I have shown above, it is not obvious that this is Descartes' view on secondary qualities. Second, the conclusions derived from (1)–(3) are very unCartesian. Descartes always lists the ideas of cold and the like among adventitious ideas or ideas of external things rather than among ideas of – so to speak – reflection.[27] It is just a fact about the phenomenology of sensations that they present themselves *as if* of external objects. And, as I argued above, even if sensations clearly and distinctly understood ought to include no more than that of which we have inner awareness (since they do not resemble anything in physical reality), our obscure and confused ideas of color still present colors as properties of bodies. Furthermore, to say that ideas of cold *represent qualia* is to contradict Descartes' doctrine of the transparency of thought;[28] for it is to say that in normal circumstances to have an idea of red is to have an

[25] Ibid., See Nelson (1996), p. 17.

[26] Ibid., p. 23.

[27] Descartes claims that ideas of color are innate in *Comments on a Certain Broadsheet*, CSM I 304; AT VIIIB 359. However, even there Descartes doesn't deny the adventitious character of these ideas. He claims that they are occasioned by corporeal motions and that we refer them to external things. Descartes does not explain why we refer them to external objects. All Descartes is concerned with, in this context, is disproving that all ideas "have their origin in observation of things" (CSM I 304; AT VIIIB 358). So, ideas of color are said to be innate insofar as they are not transmitted to us from external things and not insofar as they are perceived as coming from the mind itself. The fact that they are not transmitted to us from external things does not rule out that we perceive them *as if of* things.

[28] I am not denying that this doctrine may raise problems for Descartes vis-à-vis, for example, his doctrine of innate ideas. However, it seems that *qualia* – if anything – are the primary object of direct and transparent introspection.

idea of my feeling redly. But although Descartes would certainly not deny that we can think of our feelings, he would deny that this is what happens in normal circumstances.

2.4.2 Field's Argument

According to Richard Field, Descartes distinguishes between ideas of sense and sensations. Sensations are mere *qualia.*[29] Ideas of sense are ideas that include sensations as part of their objective content. More specifically, the idea that includes sensations as part of its objective content is the intellectual idea of body.[30] So, ideas of sense are ideas of the intellect that misrepresent sensations (or *qualia*) as modes of *res extensa.*

I disagree with Field that ideas of sense are ideas of the intellect that *contain* sensations as their objects and the nature of our disagreement will become clear in Chapters 5 and 6. Here, I just want to challenge the reasons offered by Field in support of the distinction between ideas of sense and sensations. First, according to Field, Descartes cannot claim that materially false ideas are ideas that *represent their external objects* as other than they are on pain of conflating the notions of material falsity with the notion of formal falsity. Here's how he puts it:

> Representing non things as things turns out on this proposal simply to be formal falsity, the misrepresentation of actual things, and such a misrepresentation would then be materially false if we cannot tell whether it is misrepresentation of an actual state of affairs. But as we have seen, formal falsity requires the reference of an idea to an actual state of affairs that can occur only in judgment. This account of material falsity, then, cannot account for why Descartes claims that material falsity occurs "in ideas."[31]

But this conclusion is mistaken. Ideas, according to Descartes, can be confused about the internal object being represented and this confused internal object can very well be a (possibly existing) external object and/or its properties. For example, one may believe (due to the confusion of the sensory content) that one is representing a bodily property that resembles our sensation of cold when in fact all one is representing is a

[29] See Field (1993), pp. 327–329.
[30] Ibid., p. 327.
[31] Ibid., pp. 317–318.

mode of *res extensa*. And this possibility is compatible with Descartes' view that material falsity occurs "in ideas" and is distinct from formal falsity.[32]

Second, Field claims that Descartes distinguishes ideas of sense from sensations in his replies to Arnauld. Here's the passage, from the Fourth Set of Replies, that he quotes:

> When my critic says that the idea of cold "is coldness itself in so far as it exists objectively in the intellect," I think we need to make a distinction. For it often happens in the case of obscure and confused ideas – and the ideas of heat and cold fall into this category – that an idea is referred to something other than that of which it is in fact the idea. Thus if cold is simply an absence, the idea of cold is not coldness itself as it exists objectively in the intellect, but something else, which I erroneously mistake for this absence, namely a sensation which in fact has no existence outside the intellect. (CSM II 163; AT VII 233)

Notice that Descartes could be saying either that (a) the idea of cold is the idea *of* a sensation that has no existence outside the mind (as Field reads it);[33] or that (b) the obscure and confused idea of cold *is identical with* the sensation of cold thereby claiming that the sensation itself represents (confusedly) cold as a property of body (as I, and many others, read the passage).[34] But then, given its ambiguity (and Field acknowledges this ambiguity), the above passage no more counts as evidence in support of Field's reading than against it. Moreover, (b) is a far more natural way of reading what Descartes wants to say here. Descartes is contrasting clear and distinct ideas with obscure and confused ones. And he is saying that whereas the former represent their objects as they truly are, the latter do not. They are obscure and confused representations of their objects because they represent them as other than they are ("they are referred to something other than that of

[32] Cecilia Wee also argues that Descartes' notion of material falsity ought to be kept distinct from that of formal falsity. See Wee (2006), chapter three, pp. 29–36.

[33] For a similar reading see Brown (2006), chapter four, pp. 104–109. For a reading of the notion of material falsity in Meditation Three that is also similar (at least in some respects) to Field (1993), see Vinci (1998), pp. 180–194. According to Vinci, "ideas of sense that suffer from generic material falsity are not quasi-judgmental referred sensations, but are the innate ideas of sense themselves that somehow fail to present their objects as they really are, namely as forms of sensory awareness" (Vinci (1998), p. 182).

[34] See, for example, Wilson (1978), pp. 110–114 and Kenny (1968), p. 120.

which they are in fact the ideas"). Accordingly, the idea of cold as long as it falls short of clear and distinctness, "is not coldness itself as it exists objectively in the intellect" but a sensation "which in fact has no existence outside the intellect" and, hence, represents cold as other than it truly is (that is, as a property of body resembling the felt coldness). In conclusion, Descartes is saying that the idea of cold is the same as the sensation *of* cold insofar as the "of" in "the sensation of cold" is taken as an objective genitive. Accordingly, the idea of cold does not represent the sensation but *it is* the sensation of something external which it presents as coldness.[35]

In light of 2.2–2.4 above, I conclude that there are good reasons to doubt the tenability of the non-representationalist interpretation (and its variants). And, in fact, this is the right conclusion to draw since, as I will argue next, there are both textual and theoretical reasons for believing that Descartes held that sensations are intrinsic representations of the corporeal world.

2.5 DEFEATING THE NON-REPRESENTATIONALIST INTERPRETATION

I now want to offer some positive textual evidence that Descartes believed not only that sensations of color (and the like) exhibit intrinsic intentionality but that he believed that they intrinsically represent corporeal reality.

In Meditation Three, Descartes writes that the term "idea" strictly speaking applies only to that class of thoughts that exhibit intentionality ("Some of my thoughts are as it were the images of things, and it is only in these cases that the term 'idea' is strictly appropriate" CSM II 25; AT VII 37); and that "the objective mode of being belongs to ideas by their

[35] In a passage that occurs shortly after Descartes writes: "[...] the obscurity of the idea is the only thing that leads me to judge that the idea of the sensation of cold represents some object 'cold' which is located outside me [...]" (CSM II 164; AT VII 234–235). One may argue that this passage shows quite clearly that for Descartes the idea of cold is different from the sensation of cold. However, I read it as confirming my reading that the idea of cold is the same as the sensation of cold where the "of" is to be interpreted as an objective genitive. Saying that the idea of cold represents the sensation of cold as a property of the corporeal world is the same as saying that when we sense cold we sense it as if it were a property of external things.

very nature [. . .]" (CSM II 29; AT VII 42). Interestingly, Descartes includes in the list of representative ideas perceptions of "light and colours, sounds, smells, tastes, heat and cold and the other tactile qualities" (CSM II 30; AT VII 43; see also CSM II 26; AT VII 38).

A defender of the non-representationalist interpretation may object that we should not give too much weight to the fact that Descartes calls perceptions of color and the like "ideas" because Descartes uses this term loosely as to include everything the mind is aware of (see, for example, CSM II 113; AT VII 160–161 and CSM II 253; AT VII 366). If this is the case, then sensations are rightly called "ideas" but that does not imply that they have objective being. But notice that, although Descartes does use the term "idea" as an umbrella term for different acts of the mind, in this context he is listing sensations of color and the like among ideas *after* having defined "ideas" in the strict sense of modes of thought that exhibit intentionality. And it would be very strange if, after having defined ideas in this strict sense, Descartes went back to the loose sense of "ideas" when he talks about sensations.

But the strongest evidence against the non-representationalist interpretation is provided by the notion of material falsity. According to Descartes, material falsity occurs in ideas:

> [. . .] when they represent non-things as things. For example, the ideas which I have of heat and cold contain so little clarity and distinctness that do not even enable me to tell whether cold is merely the absence of heat or vice versa, or whether both of them are real qualities, or neither is. And *since there can be no ideas which are not as it were of things*, if it is true that cold is nothing but the absence of heat, the idea which represents it to me as something real and positive deserves to be called false. (CSM II 30; AT VII 43–44, emphasis added)

First, notice that Descartes writes that sensations of color and the like are materially false ideas because they represent non-things *as* things, that is, they represent color and heat *as* something real. Since these ideas are obscure and confused we do not know, from a mere inspection of their sensory content, *what* real object they exhibit. But their representing an object to the mind – no matter how confusedly – is enough to correctly classify sensations among representative perceptions. Furthermore, according to Descartes, the something real that materially false ideas exhibit to the mind is something *external* to the mind, i.e., a yet unknown property of bodies. In Meditation Three, Descartes discusses materially false ideas in the context of his analysis of the content of ideas of "corporeal things" (CSM II 29–30; AT VII 43–44). And although the obscurity and confusion of the content of sensory ideas leads Descartes to conclude (at least, temporarily) in Meditation Three that we do not need to postulate the existence of anything else besides the mind to explain the origin of materially false ideas, Meditation Six clearly contradicts this temporary conclusion. The proof of the actual existence of material things in Meditation Six confirms, and is based on, the assumption that ideas of sense are ideas of material things.

Second, the *property of representationality* exhibited by perceptions of secondary qualities is precisely what explains the notion of material falsity. A materially false idea, according to Descartes, is an idea that provides the material for erroneous judgments about the properties of bodies (such as "The color white is in the waterlili").[36] This happens because a materially false idea represents its object *as if* it existed outside the mind; but since its representational content is obscure and confused we cannot really tell *what* this something real exhibited to the mind is; therefore, the idea may cause the erroneous judgment that there is an object outside the mind that resembles the object represented by the idea.

A supporter of the non-representationalist interpretation may concede all of this – that is, that materially false ideas exhibit intentionality and that this intentionality is responsible for the erroneous judgments based on it – but still insist that the property of representationality they exhibit isn't intrinsic to the sensation. One may argue that the property of intentionality that sensations exhibit is the result of an implicit judgment and, therefore, it is inherited.[37] In fact, a similar objection was raised by Arnauld who pointed out that the notion of material falsity conceals a confusion between ideas and judgment (CSM II 145–146; AT VII 206–207). However, I will argue in the rest of this section, that Descartes' insistence on the distinction between material and formal falsity (especially in his replies to Arnauld) is the clearest indication that Descartes did not confuse a judgment with an idea. And, so, the case of materially false ideas is indeed the best evidence that Descartes believed that sensations exhibit an intrinsic representationality prior to, and independent of, any judgment.

[36] See CSM II 163; AT VII 232.

[37] See, for example, Alanen (1994), especially p. 246.

Material falsity, writes Descartes, pertains to ideas only. More precisely, it concerns the representational content of the idea or the object the idea exhibits to the mind. Formal falsity, instead, pertains to judgments and occurs when we judge that there is an actual object that resembles the object presented by the idea (CSM II 26 and CSM II 30). Arnauld objected that "there cannot be any idea which is materially false" (CSM II 145; AT VII 206). Ideas taken in themselves, points out Arnauld, are true because the idea of cold, for example, "is coldness itself in so far as it exists in the intellect" (CSM II 145; AT VII 206). Besides, as Descartes writes in Meditation Three, "ideas, provided that they are considered in themselves and I do not refer them to anything else, they cannot strictly speaking be false" (CSM II 26; AT VII 37). So, concludes Arnauld, by calling ideas "materially false" Descartes is confusing ideas with a judgment because he is referring the idea to something else existing outside the mind.

Burman had made a similar objection. He reminded Descartes of his claim in Meditation Three that ideas themselves "simply as modes of my thought without referring them to anything else, [. . .] could *scarcely* give [us] any material for error" (CSMK 337; AT V 152, emphasis added); and then he objected to Descartes that "since all error concerning ideas comes from their relation and application to external things, there seems to be no subject matter for error whatsoever if they are not referred to externals" (CSMK 337; AT V 152).

In reply to Burman, Descartes clarifies that the notion of material falsity does not involve comparing the idea to something existing outside as follows:

> Even if I do not refer my ideas to anything outside myself, there is still subject-matter for error, since I can make a mistake with regard to the actual nature of the ideas [. . .]. For example, I may say that whiteness is a quality; and even if I do not refer this idea to anything outside myself – even if I do not say or suppose that there is any white thing – I may still make a mistake in the abstract, with regards to whiteness itself and its nature or the idea I have of it [. . .]. (CSMK 337; AT V 152)

Descartes claims here that material falsity does not depend on a comparison between the idea and something else. Rather material falsity pertains to the *internal* object of thought. Insofar as the idea presents an object to the mind and this object is only confusedly and obscurely perceived the idea is materially false because it misrepresents its object. It represents its object as other than it is and, hence, it makes a mistake "in the abstract." And by making this error in the abstract, the idea also provides the material for an erroneous judgment. For example, my experience presents the color white *as* a property of bodily surfaces (and notice that this is quite different from *believing* that whiteness is a property of bodily surfaces) and, on the basis of this experience, I may form the erroneous belief that the property of being white is a property of bodies.[38]

Descartes' replies to Arnauld also confirm that Descartes' view is that material falsity depends on the intrinsically flawed representational content of the idea. In this context, Descartes insists that it is not true that ideas taken in themselves cannot be false and the case of materially false ideas is supposed to introduce an exception. Their "falsity" is to be understood in light of the obscurity of their content:

> When my critic [Arnauld] says that the idea of cold "is coldness itself in so far as it exists objectively in the intellect", I think we need to make a distinction. For it often happens in the case of obscure and confused ideas [. . .] that an idea is referred to something other than that of which it is in fact the idea. (CSM II 164; AT VII 234)

In this passage Descartes distinguishes between clear and distinct ideas and obscure and confused ideas and clarifies that the mark of the latter is that they seem to represent what they do not in fact represent. So, the obscurity of their content explains why sensory ideas, *taken in themselves* are misrepresentations of their objects.

But the best evidence that material falsity pertains to ideas and that the representational content of sensations isn't the result of an implicit judgment comes from Descartes' explanation to Arnauld of the difference between formal and material falsity. Such a difference is illustrated in the Fourth Set of Replies in a very illuminating way. Whereas the truth value of a judgment is affected by the actual states of affairs in question (precisely because in a judgment we take the representational content of the idea to correspond to something outside the idea); the "truth value" of the representational content of an idea remains

[38] Cecilia Wee makes a similar point in Wee (2006), chapter three, pp. 29–36. According to Wee, Descartes inherits the notion of material falsity from Suarez.

unaffected by what the real object of the idea turns out to be. And this proves that the representational content of the idea isn't the result of a judgment. Here's how Descartes puts it:

> [. . .] the only sense in which an idea can be said to be "materially false" is the one which I explained [in Meditation Three]. Thus, *whether cold is a positive thing or an absence does not affect the idea I have of it, which remains the same as it always was.* (CSM II 163; AT VII 232, emphasis added)

So, Descartes insists, material falsity depends on the intrinsically flawed (because obscure and confused) representational content of the idea and this content remains totally unaffected by our discovery of what the real object of the idea is. But presumably if the representational content of the idea were the result of a judgment, then the once-materially-false ideas should turn into materially-true ones once the clear and distinct ideas of the intellect reveal to the mind what the true object of sensations is. But this, Descartes says, simply does not happen. An example may help to illustrate his point. Christopher Peacocke uses the following example to distinguish the content of experience from the judgment caused by experience: "A man may be familiar with a perfect *trompe l'oeil* violin painted on a door, and be sure from his past experience that it is a *trompe l'oeil*: nevertheless his experience may continue to represent a violin as hanging on the door in front of him."[39]

For all the above reasons, *pace* the non-representatonalist interpretation, a materially false idea, according to Descartes, is an idea that provides material for erroneous judgments in virtue of its representational content rather than exhibiting representational content in virtue of an implicit judgment.

2.6 BROADER CONSIDERATIONS

A supporter of the non-representationalist interpretation may still object that, in Meditation Six, sensations are said to represent external things because *we* implicitly judge that the ideas refer to the objects that we take to be their causes. In other words, according to this reading of Meditation Six, the explicit reasoning through which Descartes proves

[39] Peacocke (1983), p. 6. For further discussion of this see 2.6 and 5.5 below.

the existence of material things (*viz.*, that there must be a causal connection between sensory ideas and the objects they seem to represent) would in fact be the judgment that is implicitly operative in every sensation.[40] This conclusion seems to be confirmed by passages such as:

> [. . .] From the fact that I perceive by my senses a great variety of colors, sounds, smells and tastes, as well as differences in heat, hardness and the like, I am correct in *inferring* that the bodies which are the sources of these various sensory perceptions possess differences corresponding to them [. . .]. (CSM II 56; AT VII 81, emphasis added)

And in the *Passions of the Soul*, Descartes distinguishes sensations from appetites and passions as follows:

> All the perceptions [. . .] come to the soul by means of the nerves. They differ from one another in so far as *we refer* some to external objects which strike our senses [i.e., sensations], others to our body or to certain of its parts [i.e., appetites], and still others to the soul [i.e., passions in the strict sense]. (CSM I 336–337; AT XI 345, emphasis added)

> The perceptions *we refer* to things outside us, namely to the objects of our senses, are caused by these objects, at least when our judgments are not false. (CSM I 337; AT XI 346, emphasis added)

However, there are theoretical reasons why we should not conclude from either the proof in Meditation Six or the above passages that the representative character of sensations is the result of a judgment.

First, it is clear from Meditation Six that the reasoning through which Descartes explains why sensory ideas seem to represent something outside themselves (and that ultimately allows him to prove the existence of material things as the actual causes of these ideas) is not the implicit judgment that endows them with intentionality. As Descartes explains in a letter to Hyperaspistes, sensory ideas "come to us in such a way as to make us aware that they are not produced by ourselves but come from elsewhere" (CSMK 193; AT III 429) and it is precisely *this* feature of sensory ideas (i.e., that they are ideas *of* things) that generates the argument that proves the existence of material things. And, so, the

[40] For this kind of objection, see Nelson (1996).

explanation of why sensations exhibit this intrinsic world-directedness is not to be confused with the implicit judgment that would rob them of their intrinsic world-directedness.

Second, as I already anticipated in 2.3 above, I find the claim that a non-representational sensation becomes representative of some external object in virtue of act of judgment implausible. It would be agreed that there must be an explanation of *why* we make this judgment. The most natural explanation is that we judge that sensations come from the objects they represent because they *already* represent, or are of, these objects. Why would we even be led to refer (implicitly or explicitly) sensations to external objects unless sensations presented themselves *as if of* these objects?[41] But this explanation is not available to the supporter of the non-representationalist interpretation since they deny that sensations are intrinsically representational. But then, if the sensation of color (for example) presents color as a feature of my own experience why would I even be *inclined* to refer these sensations to external objects? Notice that saying that the non-representationalist interpretation is better described as holding that sensation of color and the like are *neutral* mental states, that is, mental states that present color *as* neither a property of body nor *as* a property of the mind does not help much.[42] If anything, it makes things worse. It is unclear how to understand what it means for a mental state such as the sensation of red to be neutral since that would imply that there is a prior state to the sensation *of* red (where the "of" is to be taken as an objective genitive).[43] But the phenomenology of

[41] Alison Simmons makes a similar point regarding the relation between the second and third grades of sensation in the Sixth Set of Replies: "[...] there is good reason to think that these judgments [about the size and shape of an object at the third grade of sensation] require some antecedent representation of primary qualities at the second grade. Descartes says that these spatial judgments require us to calculate one spatial quality from another (AT VII 438). We calculate size, for example, from shape and distance. In order for size to be calculated from shape and distance, however, shape and distance must already be represented to the mind. If in perceiving a fire truck, I received only a second grade sensation of unextended red, there would be no way to judge the truck's size" (Simmons (2003), p. 560).

[42] See for example, Vinci (1998), chapter seven, sections 8 and 9.

[43] Field has suggested to me, in a private exchange, that when we say that we have sensations of cold, red and so on we are merely indicating the proper classification of the sensation according to its formal being. But substituting the "of" of intentionality with the "of" of classification does not change things since sensations can still be classified in terms of their objects.

sensation excludes this possibility because sensations come to us with a built-in intentionality. The sensation of red is not experienced (in normal unreflective circumstances) as *seeing redly* but as seeing *something* red.

Another suggestion is that, according to Descartes, sensations appear to be representational in virtue of a non-volitional judgment.[44] This view is alleged to be compatible with Descartes' claims, in the Sixth Set of Replies, that the judgments at the third degree of sensation are habitual judgments (CSM II 295; AT VII 438) and his remarks that we cannot withdraw our assent from these judgments even if we know that they are mistaken (CSM II 296; AT VII 440). However, the attribution to Descartes of non-volitional judgments is problematic. Maybe we could explain these judgments in purely mechanistic terms in virtue of some principles of association along the lines of animal reasoning. But this seems to contradict Descartes' claim that habitual judgments at the third level of sensation presuppose the use of the intellect (although we may not be aware of such use). But, more importantly, the notion of non-volitional judgment is problematic in light of Descartes' view that judgments necessarily involve an act of will. For these reasons, we should avoid explaining the representational character of sensation in virtue of non-volitional judgments. My own view, as we shall see in Chapter 5 below, is that when Descartes claims that *we refer our sensations to external objects* he is not saying that this reference is the result of a non-volitional judgment but saying that *we experience external objects as colored or colors as properties of objects.* A similar view can be found in Brown (2006):

> It is useful at this point to compare the function of "referring" in Descartes' epistemology to the notion of "seeing as" in contemporary analyses of perception. Could we say, for example, that to refer a sensation of whiteness to the paper is analogous to seeing the paper as white? To refer pain to the foot is to feel the foot as afflicted [...]. Such locutions represent an object, for example, [...] the foot, as being modified in a certain way [...]. One advantage of the seeing-as talk over talk of judgments is that it enables one to ascribe structured representational content to a perception without collapsing the distinction between perception and belief or judgment. [...] The seeing-as locution is

[44] On this see Simmons (2003), especially pp. 563–575. Lilli Alanen seems to hint at this possible position in a footnote, but she does not explicitly argue for it. See Alanen (1994), p. 246, fn. 30.

preferable, in my view, to the terminology of judgment, for the reason that judgment and acts of assent are generally connected in Descartes' framework.[45]

I agree with Brown's claim that the perceiving-as locution allows us to talk of *structured experiential content* without collapsing the distinction between the content of experience and the beliefs caused by that content. In fact, I believe that acknowledging the notion of a structured experiential content such as perceiving *x* as *y* is the necessary intermediate step between sensory experience and sensory based beliefs and judgments.[46] After all, Descartes does say of the perceptions with which we refer to our body that "we *feel* [as opposed to *judge*] [them] as being in our limbs" (CSM I 337; AT XI 346–347). Likewise, we *sense* colors *as* being in things outside us.[47]

There is another broad reason why we ought to believe that Descartes attributed intrinsic intentionality to sensations. As Martial Gueroult and Marjorie Grene have brought to our attention, Descartes' own method of inquiry testifies that ideas are the basic units of knowledge. What Descartes is after is "not judgments like those of Aristotle and Kant, but a series of entirely reliable mental acts that carry me by their very nature to trust the veridicality of their contents."[48] Think of how the meditator is invited to search for truth. After the doubts of Meditation One and the discovery of the first truth in Meditation Two, Descartes, in Meditation Three, proceeds to enumerate various ideas within himself in order to investigate whether any of them *in virtue of its*

[45] Brown (2006), p. 101.

[46] These issues will be discussed again in 5.5 below. Brown and I differ, however, in how to explain the notion of perceiving-as within Descartes' philosophy. Brown, as far as I can tell, leaves the notion unaccounted for. See especially Brown (2006), pp. 94–109.

[47] One could argue that the structured experiential content is itself the result of a referral judgment made in infancy. See, for example, Vinci (1998), chapter four, especially 4.3–4.5. According to Vinci, "erroneous" experiential contents are the result of what he calls "immature referrals" (Ibid., p. 132). Immature referrals are made in infancy in virtue of a psychophysical mechanism that operates according to a resemblance principle that makes "the physiological system" (Ibid., p. 135) hypothesize that the world is exactly like the felt sensations. Vinci's claim is based on reading Principles I.71 as suggesting that there is a stage in infancy when pure sensations are distinguished from the perception of the physical world. As we shall see in Chapter 6 below, I disagree with the above reading of Principles I.71. Besides, it is not obvious that the "physiological system" could refer sensations to the external world in purely mechanistic terms. Vinci's explanation is sketchy and unsupported textually (see, Ibid., pp. 134–135).

[48] Grene (1985), p. 6.

very content gives sufficient ground to infer the existence of anything else besides the self. It is in this context that Descartes makes a distinction between confused and obscure ideas, on the one hand, and clear and distinct ideas, on the other. A clear and distinct idea is an idea whose content is not only accessible to the mind but also is a reliable presentation of its object (See CSM II 31–32; AT VII 46 and CSM I 207–208; AT VIIIA 22). As such, a clear and distinct idea "can serve as the basis for a certain and indubitable judgment" (CSM I 207; AT VIIIA 21–22 and CSM II 37–43; AT VII 53–62). On the contrary, it is the lack of perspicuity and distinctness of the content of sensory ideas that makes them the subject matter for false judgments (CSM II 30; AT VII 44; CSM II 163; AT VII 232–234). So, only clear and distinct ideas are such that they exhibit their objective reality on their sleeves and, therefore, can be trusted to infer the possible existence of their objects. Ideas of sense are obscure and confused and it is this feature that does not allow us (or ought not to allow us) to infer the possible existence of the objects obscurely represented.[49] And the whole point of Descartes' method consists in analyzing the content of ideas in order to identify the clear elements (or simple notions) in their contents and, hence, avoid making mistaken judgments on the basis of confused contents (see CSM I 208; AT VIIIA 22). As Grene puts it, Descartes' search for knowledge consists in the examination "within [. . .] ideas for their clarity and distinctness and in particular for their degree of objective reality."[50] So, Descartes' own method for searching after truth seems to provide indirect evidence that, according to him, ideas and their contents (be they clear and distinct or obscure and confused) are the basic units of knowledge upon which judgment is based. Accordingly,

[49] Notice that, in the Fourth Set of Replies, Descartes classifies ideas as more or less materially false depending on the degree of obscurity of their content (CSM II 163–164; AT VII 233–234). "Ideas which give the judgment little or no scope for error" writes Descartes, "do not seem as much entitled to be called materially false as those which give great scope for error" (CSM II 163; AT VII 233). And the greatest scope for error is provided by the confused ideas of the senses. Why? Because, explains Descartes, "the obscurity of the idea is the only thing that leads me to judge that the idea of the sensation of cold represents some object called 'cold' which is located outside of me" (CSM II 164; AT VII 234).

[50] Grene (1985), p. 17.

Descartes' view is that judgments must conform to the ways in which we perceive objects through our ideas rather than being the reason why we perceive objects through ideas.

Finally, a representationalist interpretation explains why, according to Descartes, sensations have both a cognitive and pragmatic role. According to Descartes, sensations contain some truth (CSM II 56; AT VII 80), that is, they provide a partially correct representation of things. And their representation is partially correct because sensations inform us of the presence of external objects despite the fact that they misrepresent these objects and their properties. This "truthfulness" explains both why sensations have the pragmatic role of preserving the well-being of the mind–body union and why the senses are part of the same search after truth as the intellect. The senses, according to Descartes, provide us with information that is the starting point of a scientific inquiry that culminates with clear and distinct perception. But if sensations were mere ornaments of the mind it would be difficult to see how they could be used either for survival or as the starting point of a scientific inquiry continuous with that of the intellect.

CONCLUSION

Sections 2.2–2.4 show that neither a sound argument nor incontrovertible textual evidence supports the non-representationalist interpretation. Sections 2.5–2.6 provide reasons for believing the opposite, that is, that Descartes attributed intrinsic intentionality to sensations. I conclude that the non-representationalist interpretation is *not* the correct interpretation of Cartesian sensations and, hence, that the exegetical and theoretical puzzle of sensory representation is *not* a red herring. I now turn to discussing various representationalist accounts of Cartesian sensations and the solutions to the puzzle that stem from them.

3

Externalist Solutions: Causal Accounts

Two different types of representationalism about Cartesian sensations can be found in the literature, i.e., externalism and internalism. Externalism comes in two varieties – causal and teleofunctional. In this chapter, I will discuss the former. Despite the considerable agreement in the literature that bodies play some causal role in Descartes' account of sensation, only a few scholars have developed this claim into a full-fledged causal account of the representationality of Cartesian sensations (CA).[1] The most prominent defenders, and self-declared representatives, of this view are Margaret Wilson and Tad Schmaltz.[2] Since I take Wilson and Schmaltz to have laid out the groundwork for causal accounts of Cartesian sensations, I will make their views the primary focus of this chapter.

As we shall see, the main motivation for, and advantage of, CA consists in providing an easy solution to the problem of sensory misrepresentation.[3] However, *contra* both Wilson and Schmaltz, I argue that causal accounts fail to explain both the representationality of Cartesian sensations and the puzzle of sensory representation. I conclude that these failures

[1] Many scholars have defended the claim that bodies are causes (as opposed to mere occasions) of ideas of sense in the context of the debate on whether Descartes' doctrine of the innateness of ideas of sense commits him necessarily to occasionalism. However, such defense (by and large) does not extend to the stronger claim that bodies are the causes of the representational content of sensory ideas. See for example, Kenny (1968); McRae (1972); Adams (1975); Clarke (1982); Cottingham (1986); Jolley (1990); Wilson (1991); Garber (1993); Nadler (1994); Rozemond (1999); Schmaltz (1997); Scott (2000) and Kendrick (2000). For the denial that bodies are causes of sensory ideas, see Broughton (1986) and Gorham (2002).

[2] See Wilson (1990) and Schmaltz (1992). Hoffman (1996), Normore (1986) and, to a certain extent, De Rosa (2004) are also sympathetic to causal accounts.

[3] This is particularly explicit in Wilson (1990).

indicate that an internalist element (along the lines of DA) *must* be present even in Descartes' account of sensory representation. This conclusion is the theoretical foundation of the alternative reading of the representationality of sensations that I will defend in Chapter 5.

3.1 GENERAL FEATURES OF CA

Before we plunge into a discussion of the details of Wilson's and Schmaltz's accounts, I want to highlight some general features that they share *qua* causal accounts. First, both accounts challenge the claim that *representationality* is an internal property of sensory ideas by arguing that these ideas represent what they do in virtue of a causal relation with their right objects. That is, *contra* internalist interpretations, Descartes would be committed to a relational reading of the objective reality of ideas according to which ideas represent their right objects in virtue of a mind–world relation.

Second, the claim that sensory ideas represent what they do in virtue of a causal relation implies a different reading of Descartes' claim that *an idea of x is just x itself as it exists in the understanding* (CSM II 75; AT VII 102) and, hence, of the claim that there is a correspondence between the presentational and referential content of an idea. As we shall see, the causal interpretation of the above claim is the mirror image (so to speak) of its internalist interpretation. According to an internalist interpretation, an idea cannot but *referentially* represent what it presentationally represents because the presentational content determines the referential content; conversely, according to a causal interpretation, an idea cannot but *presentationally* represent what it referentially represents because the idea presentationally and referentially represents what causes it.[4]

Third, causal accounts render the notion of referential representation pivotal in Descartes' theory of ideas. If ideas are individuated by their objective reality and what determines the objective reality of ideas is a causal connection with their right object (referent), then the notion of referential representation becomes the most important sense of representation within Descartes' theory of ideas. It is necessary to highlight this feature because it

[4] Only Paul Hoffman seems to be aware of this implication and the potential problem that it raises for explaining sensory misrepresentation. See Hoffman (1996), p. 366. I will return to this below.

is something that causal theorists underplay. And although it would be question begging to deny that Descartes held this view without first looking at the arguments by which causal theorists attribute it to Descartes, we should keep this consequence of their reading in mind in evaluating the overall tenability of causal accounts.

Finally, there are at least two different ways of explaining misrepresentation and they depend crucially on how we take the phrase *they represent their objects* in the sentence "they represent their objects as other than they are." As we saw in Chapters 1 and 2, I take these objects to be modes of *res extensa.* But even assuming that these objects are modes of *res extensa* we can take the phrase "they represent their objects" either *de re* or *de dicto.* According to a *de re* reading, the phrase means *they stand for (or refer to) modes of* res extensa (independently of any description associated with the idea and in virtue of a causal connection). According to a *de dicto* reading, the phrase means *they present (or describe) modes of* res extensa.[5] As we shall see, causal accounts explain misrepresentation on the basis of a *de re* reading.

After highlighting the general features of causal readings, we can proceed to our discussion of the details of Wilson's and Schmaltz's accounts.

3.2 WILSON'S CA

Wilson proposes a new way of dealing with the problem of sensory misrepresentation. Rather than concluding that Descartes' overall internalist account of ideas is evidence that the case of materially false ideas is at best a confusion between ideas and judgments (as Arnauld and many others are inclined to believe) Wilson argues that the case of materially false ideas is evidence that Descartes did *not* have an overall internalist account of ideas. In the case of sensory representation, according to Wilson, Descartes thought that the presentational and referential senses of representation come apart. They are distinct from, and independent of, one another and this distinction accounts for the very possibility of misrepresentation. Here's how Wilson puts it:

[5] For the distinction between *de dicto* and *de re* ascriptions see, for example, Richard (1997), p. 214: "*De dicto* ascriptions report that the believer has what a sentence says – a *dictum*, or proposition – as the object of an attitude. *De re* ascriptions relate the believer to a thing (or *res*) [...] specified independently of how the believer conceptualizes it."

[...] the representationality of ideas does consist *partly* in presentational content. However, an idea's [...] representing n does not preclude that the idea presents n as other than it is. [...] Descartes' notion of representation [is] partly "referential", as a way of expressing the non-presentational element.[6]

In the above passage, Wilson writes that the notion of referential content, in the case of sensory ideas, ought to be understood "as a way of expressing the non-presentational element." I take it to mean that she attributes to Descartes the view that the referential content of the idea is determined independently of its presentational content. This is confirmed by the following passage:

In view of some recent theories of reference and perception, one might hope for a causal account of "referential" or non-presentational representation: an idea, that is, referentially represents its cause (or cause under normal conditions), whatever that might be. Thus, for my idea of cold referentially to represent a certain physical state is just for that idea to be caused – in the "right" way – by that state, whatever that may be.[7]

The referential content of ideas, then, according to Wilson's Descartes, is determined relationally (*viz.*, by a causal relation with the environment) as opposed to being determined by the presentational content of the idea (*viz.*, by a description of the object associated with the idea). This conclusion is *forced on us*, argues Wilson, because if the referential content were determined by the presentational content (along the lines of DA), we could not explain material falsity (or sensory misrepresentation), as Arnauld pointed out.

The Cartesian notion of presentational content would then play the secondary role of providing a mere description of how the object appears to me (quite independently of how the object actually is):

Roughly [presentational representation] coincides with what the mind takes itself to be aware of (If I think I see a tanager, then I can be ascribed a presentational representation of a tanager, regardless of what may actually be going on in the world [...])[8]

6 Wilson (1990), reprinted in Wilson (1999), p. 73.
7 Ibid., p. 75.
8 Ibid., p. 81, fn. 10.

Notice, in passing, that this notion of presentational content is less than clear. All that is clear is that presentational content, according to Wilson, plays no role whatsoever in fixing the right object of sensory ideas (or their objective reality). But here are some questions that deserve an answer and receive none in Wilson's account. Does presentational content amount to the purely subjective and qualitative aspect of experience? This does not seem to be the case for, in the above quotation, Wilson claims that it consists in the presentation *of an object* to the mind. But then, what object is it presenting to the mind? Is it presenting to the mind the *same object* that is referentially represented? If yes, how does that happen? Moreover, if the presentational content consists in the presentation of an object to the mind, where does the intentionality of the idea come from? Is that an internal feature of the idea? This seems to follow from the fact that presentational content is introduced as a non-relational feature of content. But can ideas, in virtue of some internal feature, present a *particular* object, i.e., a tanager? I will return to these questions below. For the time being, let me continue to summarize Wilson's views.

At times, Wilson seems to understand Descartes' notions of presentational and referential representations along the lines of what nowadays would be called – respectively – narrow and wide contents. Wide contents are individuated relationally in virtue of a causal relation with the environment; narrow contents are individuated non-relationally. And along the lines of contemporary two-factor theories of content, Wilson attributes to Descartes the view that wide content (the referent) is not determined by narrow content (presentational content). This way of understanding the relation between presentational and referential content is confirmed by the (only) example she provides to illustrate the notions. According to this view, Wilson writes, "being an idea of x" is ambiguous between a *referential* and a *presentational* reading. Suppose the mind is an immaterial substance but I believe it is material. So, my idea of the mind represents an immaterial substance (in the referential sense), though it represents it to me as a material substance (in the presentational sense). Misrepresentation is then explained by the mismatch between presentational and referential content.

Wilson finds textual support for her interpretation in Descartes' replies to Arnauld. In response to Arnauld's claim that the idea of cold is coldness itself insofar as it exists objectively in the understanding, Descartes urges the necessity of distinguishing clear and distinct ideas from the obscure and confused ideas of sense:

[...] we need to make a distinction. For it often happens in the case of obscure and confused ideas [...] that an idea is referred to something other than that of which it is in fact an idea (*ut ad aliud referantur quam ad id cuius revera ideae sunt*). Thus if cold is simply an absence, the idea of cold is not coldness itself as it exists objectively in the intellect, but something else, which I erroneously mistake for this absence, namely a sensation which in fact has no existence outside the intellect. (CSM II 163; AT VII 233)

Descartes indicates that we need to draw a distinction between ideas whose presentational content is obscure and confused (sensory ideas) and ideas whose content is clear and distinct (the ideas of the intellect). Only in the latter case, Descartes claims, presentational and referential content correspond (so as to suggest that the former determines the latter along the lines of DA). But in the former case the situation is different. The idea of cold represents its object (i.e., coldness, whatever it turns out to be) as other than it is (as resembling the sensation). The important thing to notice, argues Wilson, is that Descartes, even under the pressure of Arnauld's criticism, sticks to his view that the idea of cold is still the idea *of* cold even if cold does not resemble the sensation of cold. Here's how Descartes, according to Wilson, puts it in the above passage. He claims that the idea of cold *is a sensation that presents something (or is referred to something, "referantur") other than that of which it is in fact an idea (cold as it is in nature).*[9] So, Descartes believes that the idea of cold can provide a false presentation of that of which it is in fact the idea (the mode of *res extensa* that does not resemble the idea) *while remaining the idea of cold* (*contra* what Arnauld had argued). Wilson's reasoning is that Descartes could have maintained this only if he thought that an idea can refer to its object independently of the way in which the object is presented to the mind, or *de re.* In other words, the *only* possibility of describing the idea of cold as a misrepresentation of its true object (i.e., coldness as it is in nature) depends, according to Wilson, *on this referential sense of representation.* It depends on the possibility of saying *of* cold that it is something else. So, Wilson concludes, Descartes rejects Arnauld's claim that if the idea of cold presents

[9] The reading of the above passage depends on the interpretation of the meaning of the verb "refero." In Latin, "refero" means "to report" and hence it seems closer in meaning to "to present" than to "to refer" (in the sense in which referring and reference, in philosophy of language and mind, are opposed to describing).

cold as something positive it is not the idea of cold and, hence, defends his notion of material falsity. The above passage suggests, then, that we should distinguish between what the idea *presents* to the mind and what the idea *referentially* represents. A distinction between these two senses of "representation" seems required since what the idea (referentially) represents is *not* determined by what it (presentationally) represents. And since an idea may referentially represent *n* but presentationally represent *n* as other than *n* is, the idea misrepresents its "correct" object and provides the material for error.[10]

Although highly influential, Wilson's causal account of Cartesian sensations is also highly sketchy. Wilson admits that neither Descartes nor she on Descartes' behalf "develop [the causal account] fully, to create a theory immune to counter-examples."[11] Moreover, Wilson never identifies any Cartesian doctrine that may support the causal reading. To the contrary, she admits that this reading may be difficult to reconcile, for example, with the Cartesian claim that "non-existents can be referentially represented" (implying that a non-existent can be "referentially represented" only through its presentational content, *contra* the causal reading of referential representation).[12] In conclusion, Wilson proposes this causal reading mostly on "in principle" reasons. As she puts it, attributing the causal account of sensation to Descartes, "seems necessary to make good sense of his response to Arnauld's objection"[13] where he defends the notion of materially false ideas.

So, even assuming that Wilson's intuitions are correct, a basic question remains unanswered: if there is room for a causal element in Descartes' account of the representationality of sensations, where is this room to be found? In which Cartesian doctrine? As we shall see below, one of Schmaltz's main contributions to the literature consists in identifying this doctrine in Descartes' causal principles. But before we move on, I want to examine more closely the implications of, and the problems raised by, Wilson's attribution of a causal account of sensory representation and misrepresentation to Descartes.

[10] Whether this reading is actually supported by the above passage is contentious. I believe that, even if this is a possible reading of the text, it is certainly not an obvious one.
[11] Wilson (1990), reprinted in Wilson (1999), p. 76.
[12] Ibid., p. 76 and fns 14 and 15.
[13] Ibid., p. 76.

3.3 PROBLEMS WITH WILSON'S CA

In this section, I raise four problems ((a)–(d)) for Wilson's CA. As we shall see later on, Schmaltz's CA differs in relevant respects from Wilson's and, so, these problems will apply to his account slightly differently. This is the reason why I discuss the two accounts and their respective difficulties separately so as to give the reader a better sense of some of the variations within causal accounts rather than collapsing them all in one monolithic theory.

3.3.1 (a) Is Objective Reality a Relational Notion for Descartes?

I start by highlighting a textual difficulty that Wilson only hints at but fails to deal with. Curiously, this textual issue is not, by and large, discussed by critics of causal accounts.[14] According to Wilson's Descartes, the objective reality of sensory ideas is determined by a mind–world relation. Ideas can be said to "*represent their (right) objects* as other than they are" because they are caused by them in the right way. And since the Cartesian notion of objective reality is related to the representation (I am using this term neutrally here) of the right object, according to Wilson, the objective reality of sensory ideas is determined by a causal relation.

Simply denying that Descartes held this account of objective reality on the basis of the "internalist" reading of this notion offered in Chapter 1 would beg the question with Wilson. For her argument is that the notion of material falsity *forces* us to surrender the internalist reading of objective reality in the case of sensory ideas. But, first, even if Wilson were right, we should not be so quick to dismiss all those passages where Descartes denies that ideas represent what they do in virtue of a relation with the actually existing objects being represented.[15] At the very least, an explanation ought to be provided as to how to reconcile these passages with a causal account. However, no such explanation is provided by

[14] Simmons (1999), for example, criticizes causal accounts but does not raise this textual issue.

[15] For some of these passages see 1.1 above.

Wilson. Second, I want to reconsider her argument that we *must* attribute a causal theory to Descartes on pain of not being able to explain why sensory ideas represent their objects as other than they are. *Contra* Wilson, there is an alternative way of explaining why sensory ideas represent their right objects as other than they are that does not invoke a causal account and is along the lines of DA.[16]

As we saw above, Wilson claims that the *only* way to explain why sensory ideas represent their *right* objects as other than they are consists in interpreting the phrase "represent their *right* objects" *de re*. But we can take the phrase "represent their *right* objects" *de dicto* and explain misrepresentation equally well, roughly, as follows.[17] In sensory representation the phenomenological aspect of sensory experience is mixed up with the world-directedness of the sensory idea (due, for instance, to the latent presence of the intellectual ideas of extension and figure) and, so, we confusedly (presentationally) represent the (true) object of the idea (i.e., a mode of *res extensa*) as resembling the sensation. But once we clarify the sensory content in light of the clear and distinct ideas of the intellect, we can see that what sensory ideas truly (presentationally) represent are bodies that do not resemble the sensation. So, sensory ideas represent their objects as other than they are because they *present* the (true) object of thought obscurely and confusedly. Notice that no *referential* sense of representation is invoked here to explain misrepresentation.

Moreover, this alternative explanation is compatible with a passage from Descartes' Fourth Set of Replies which creates a problem for Wilson's interpretation. As we saw above, Arnauld had objected that the notion of material falsity is incoherent because it is inconsistent with Descartes' DA. Accordingly, he protested: "What does the idea of cold, which you say is materially false represent to your mind? An absence? But in that case it is true. A positive entity? But in that case it is not the

[16] I find the model of this alternative explanation in Bolton (1986). However, as we shall see in Chapter 5, my positive account of sensory representation ends up being quite different from Bolton's. My understanding of Bolton's position has also benefited from numerous conversations with her and from reading her unpublished manuscript in English "The work of Margaret Wilson: a Talk for the APA." The work is currently published in Spanish. See Bolton (2002).

[17] A detailed explanation of my understanding of the mechanisms of misrepresentation along similar lines will be provided in Chapter 5 below.

idea of cold" (CSM II 145; AT VII 206). Descartes replies in a way which is at odds with Wilson's interpretation. He responds to Arnauld:

> *That is right* (*Recte*). But my only reason for calling an idea materially false is that owing to the fact that it is obscure and confused, I am unable to judge whether or not what it represents to me is something positive which exists outside of my sensation. (CSM II 164; AT VII 234, emphasis added)

If Wilson's interpretation were right, Descartes ought to have simply denied the assumptions that drive Arnauld's objection rather than agreeing with them (as the *Recte* confirms). Wilson, in order to defend her interpretation, dismisses this part of Descartes' reply to Arnauld by claiming that "he merely expressed himself ineptly."[18] But the alternative interpretation of material falsity offered above can easily explain Descartes' answer to Arnauld. His response confirms that he is *not* (at least not completely) abandoning DA. Rather, Descartes focuses on the distinction between *the obscure and confused* and the *clear and distinct* presentations of objects and explains misrepresentation as a case of obscure and confused *presentation* of the object of thought.[19]

3.3.2 (b) Is Misrepresentation Explained?

A second problem with Wilson's causal account – which has not been discussed in the literature – consists in whether it can explain the phenomenon of misrepresentation. According to her account, an idea is an idea *of* n *because it is caused by ns* in the right way. But notoriously, causal theories have difficulties explaining misrepresentation.[20] According to a causal

[18] Wilson (1990), reprinted in Wilson (1999) p. 75. I was also wrong in dismissing this textual evidence in De Rosa (2004).

[19] One could suggest that Descartes is agreeing with Arnauld ("*Recte*") only on the assumption that materially false ideas are representational; but that he concludes with a denial of this assumption ("But my only reason for calling an idea materially false is that [...] it is obscure and confused"). However, I disagree with this reading of the text for Descartes writes that a materially false idea is obscure and confused insofar as "I am unable to judge whether or not *what it represents to me* is something positive which exists outside of my sensation."

[20] See, for example, Fodor (1987) and Fodor (1990). Here I am discussing what in the literature are known as "historical" or "crude" causal theories (that is, theories according to which concepts represent what actually or historically causes them) since Wilson seems to be thinking of causal theories in historical rather than counterfactual terms.

theory, the idea *represents* what actually causes it. So, for example, if a causal connection with cows is a necessary condition for determining the content of the idea of cow, the idea of cow refers to cows and represents them *as* cows. Perceptual error and misrepresentation seem to be impossible. Jerry Fodor, for example, presents the difficulty as follows:

> Suppose, for example, that tokenings of the symbol "A" are nomologically dependent upon instantiations of the property A; viz., upon A's. Then according to the theory the tokens of the symbol denote A's (since tokens denote their causes) and *they represent them as A's (since symbols express the property whose instantiations cause them to be tokened). But symbol tokenings that represent A's as A's are ipso facto veridical.* So it seems that the condition for an "A"-token meaning A is identical to the condition for such a token being true. How then do you get *un*veridical "A" tokens into the causal picture?[21]

Now, let's take the idea of red. According to a causal theory, the idea of red is the idea of the property of being red (i.e., a mode of *res extensa*) because it is caused by it in the right way. But then either the idea of red represents the property of being red as it is (i.e., as a mode of *res extensa*) and so it is "true"; or if it represents it as other than it is (i.e., as other than a mode of *res extensa*), it is *not* the idea *of* red (since the idea cannot but *present* what causes it).[22] Either way, there is no room for misrepresentation. And so CA does not fare any better than DA in accounting for misrepresentation. In fact, it seems to suffer from the *mirror image* of the same problem, as we anticipated in section 3.1 above.[23]

One may object that this is an unfair reading of Wilson's account because it assumes that an idea expresses the property whose instantiations reliably cause it. But Wilson has the resources to deny this assumption by endorsing a two-factor theory of content, according to which the presentational content of an idea (roughly, what the object appears to be to us) is independent of its referential content (what the object of the idea actually is). According to Wilson, one may insist,

[21] Fodor (1987), p. 101, emphasis added.

[22] An idea is the idea *of* red because it is caused by the property of being red (a particular mode of *res extensa*); an idea expresses the property that causes it; so, if the idea of red expresses a property other than a mode of *res extensa* (for example, a property resembling the sensation), it is not the idea *of* red.

[23] I will discuss Paul Hoffman's and Tad Schmaltz's possible answers to this difficulty below.

it is precisely in virtue of this distinction that we can explain why an idea misrepresents its object. For the object presentationally represented to the mind need not be the same as the actual object the idea refers to.

This is a fair response to my criticism. But it only makes things worse for it is not clear how we can explain the phenomenon of misrepresentation once presentational and referential contents are pried apart in this way (at least if we assume with Wilson that misrepresentation is a feature intrinsic to the idea rather than being the result of a judgment). As I pointed out above, Wilson does not say much about presentational content but from the only example she provides we can evince that she intends it to be intentional. Now, let's assume that this intentionality is internal to the idea (since this assumption would allow Wilson to circumvent my previous criticism). Then, there are other serious difficulties. First, it is unclear how the intentionality of the presentational content can be explained internally, on Wilson's account. She simply does not address this question. Secondly, and more importantly, although the presentational and referential content may represent two different objects, in order for the idea to count as a misrepresentation of its object it must be the case, *minimally*, that what the idea presentationally represents "relates to" what it referentially represents (on pain of making misrepresentation the result of a wrong judgment that *we* make). But once we attribute to Wilson this "schizophrenic" account of content, it becomes difficult to explain how the presentational and referential contents stay in sync in a way that allows us to explain misrepresentation as a mismatch between them. Both claiming that it is the internal feature of the presentational content that helps us track the referent of the idea and claiming that it is the referent of the idea that determines the presentational content of the idea would violate the assumption that these two contents are independent of (and distinct from) one another. At best, then, the harmony between presentational and referential content is a mystery and, then, the mechanism of misrepresentation remains unexplained.

I conclude that if presentational and referential contents are pried apart the phenomenon of misrepresentation becomes insurmountable. Either the harmony between presentational and referential content is a mystery and, hence, the mechanism of misrepresentation remains unexplained or we can explain why presentational and referential contents represent the same object but then they cannot be regarded as two *distinct* factors (and then the threat of problem (b) is re-introduced).[24]

3.3.3 (c) Causation and Representationality?

It is questionable whether a causal connection is sufficient to explain the *representationality* of sensation. How can effects *inherently* represent their causes? Why would a causal link with an object be sufficient to explain the *representation of* that object? After all, the commotion of microscopic particles in the fire causes a piece of wax to melt but we would not say that the melting of the wax represents the commotion of particles. Short of believing in the reality of secondary qualities and in a resemblance theory of perception, how can we explain the fact that a particular configuration of particles causally linked with my mind produces a sensation that represents that cause? It may be suggested that *we* take the sensation as a *sign* of the cause. In other words, *our intentions* would translate the effect into a full-fledged representation. But this is neither what a causal theory claims nor what Wilson claims and, so, this is not an answer to the above question.[25] The problem remains and is quite pressing.[26]

As we shall see below, Schmaltz's account provides a possible solution to this objection. Unfortunately, however, I will argue that this solution undermines CA since it reintroduces through the back door the necessity of an internalist element in Descartes' account of sensory representation.

[24] Catherine Wilson, in a private exchange, has suggested to me that, according to Margaret Wilson, the "presentational content" associated to sensory ideas consists in a false *theory* of what the referent is. If this is what Wilson (1990) meant (and I am not sure that it is), then it would complicate things further. This view would imply that the referent of sensory ideas is determined both by a theory (and by a false theory as well as by a true theory, presumably) and by a causal connection.

[25] Besides, there are both textual and philosophical reasons for denying that Descartes held the view that sensations are natural signs of their effects. This reading of Descartes has been defended by Yolton (1984) and, more recently (and in a qualified way), by Chignell (2009). For further discussion of this kind of reading see 6.3 below.

[26] For a similar point see Simmons (1999), p. 353; and Pessin (2009). Richard Field, in a private exchange, expressed similar worries about causal accounts.

3.3.4 (d) The Qua-Problem

Not only is CA insufficient to explain how the causal action of *x* on the mind becomes a *representation* of *x*, but it is also insufficient to explain why the sensation is a representation of *x* as opposed to a representation of *y*, where *x* and *y* are both causally linked to the mind experiencing the sensation. For example, the simple causal connection with a body fails to explain why we take the cause of the idea to be a body (i.e., the distal cause) as opposed to a brain state (i.e., the proximate cause) where both are causes of the idea. So, CA is insufficient to fix the object of the representation. But that's exactly what it is supposed to do.

As a general criticism to simple causal theories of content this point was made by Kim Sterelny and Michael Devitt and is known in the contemporary literature as the "*qua* problem."[27] The problem can be summarized as follows. According to a simple causal theory, the idea of cat refers to cats because it is caused by cats in normal circumstances. But cats are also animals, vertebrates and so on. So, why is the concept caused by cat-or-animal-or-vertebrate the concept *of cat* rather than the concept *of animal* or *of vertebrate*? The conclusion drawn by Sterelny is that there must be *something* else that determines that it is *qua* cats that these animals caused the concept. And the "qua problem" consists precisely in explaining what is this something that determines which one of the many causes of an idea is the one that fixes its referent. The conclusion to be drawn is that *at best* a causal account needs to be complemented by a different account of how the object of the idea is fixed. But, then, it remains to be seen whether a causal theory so complemented still counts as a *causal* account. I will address this question below and then in Chapters 4 and 5.

Alison Simmons raised a similar problem for CA:

> The simple causal theory fails to isolate in a principled way the distal cause as the proper *res repraesentata* of a sensation: many things cause the sensation; including a variety of things intervening between the distal cause and the sensation (motions in the medium, changes in sensory physiology, a pattern traced on the retina of the pineal gland). Why shouldn't these intervening

[27] See Sterelny (1983) and Devitt & Sterelny (1987).

causes have as much right as the distal cause to be the sensation's *res repraesentata*?[28]

Notice that problems (c) and (d) relate to problem (a) insofar as they challenge the claim that the objective reality of sensory ideas is determined causally.

3.4 SCHMALTZ'S CA

One of the merits of Schmaltz's account consists in identifying the causal principles of Meditation Three and their employment in the proof of the existence of material things in Meditation Six as, respectively, the Cartesian doctrine and textual evidence that support the attribution of CA to Descartes. A brief digression on the causal principles of Meditation Three and Schmaltz's reading of them is then in order. Schmaltz (1992) interprets the causal principle of Meditation Three as a "Containment principle" such that:

> An efficient cause must contain either formally or eminently all the perfections or properties contained in its effect.[29]

According to Descartes, an object *contains a property formally* if that property exists in the object in a way that "*exactly corresponds to our perception of it*" (CSM II 114; AT VII 161); and an object contains a property eminently if that property exists in the object in a way that does not exactly correspond to our perception of it because it exists in the objects in a higher form (CSM II 114; AT VII 161). From the above definitions of formal and eminent containment it follows, according to Schmaltz, that we ought to read the Containment Principle as implying that:

[28] Simmons (1999), p. 353. Simmons, on the basis of this criticism, argues that the proper *res repraesentata* of a sensation is not fixed by a causal connection but by the biological function of sensations. But she is clear that the cost of supplementing a causal account of the representationality of sensation with a teleofunctional one amounts to abandoning a causal account. And she is certainly entitled to this conclusion since what fixes the object of the sensation is the biological function of the sensation. I will discuss Simmons' views in Chapter 4 below.

[29] See Schmaltz (1992), p. 40.

An efficient cause must either contain the same properties as its effect (as the notion of formal containment dictates) or contain those properties in a higher form (according to the notion of eminent containment).[30]

For our purposes we can leave aside the notion of eminent containment and focus on that of formal containment.[31] Schmaltz calls the part of the Containment principle that deals with the notion of formal containment the "Formal Containment Principle." This principle when applied to the objective reality of ideas is called "The Objective Reality Principle" and it can be phrased as follows:

X (where x is a body or a property of bodies) is the efficient cause of the objective reality of ideas only if x contains the same properties as those contained objectively in the idea.[32]

Notice the strong *similarity condition* imposed on causation in all the various versions of the formal containment principle. Against those scholars who have argued that this similarity condition precludes body-to-mind causation, Schmaltz's bold and innovative move consists

[30] Notice, however, that it does not seem to follow from the definition of formal containment provided by Descartes (an object contains a property formally if that property exists in the object in a way that "exactly corresponds to our perception of it" CSM II 114; AT VII 161) that cause and effect must have the same nature. I am assuming here that the inference is valid for the sake of argument.

[31] Again, I am assuming here with Schmaltz and O'Neill (see O'Neill (1987)) that Descartes' view is that bodies do not contain any properties eminently and, therefore, cannot be eminent causes of sensory ideas. However, this claim could be contested. The claim is based on the following reasoning: a cause contains the properties of the effect eminently only if the cause is higher on the ontological scale than the effect; but bodies are not higher on the ontological scale than minds because bodies contain the property of extension; the property of extension is an imperfection and, therefore, bodies are less perfect and lower on the ontological scale than minds. However, this reasoning can be challenged on at least two different grounds. First, it is based on a very specific reading of the notion of eminent containment and given the obscurity of the notion it is questionable whether this is exactly what Descartes had in mind. On a different reading of eminent containment, according to which, a cause is said to contain the property of the effect eminently when it can cause the effect without instantiating its properties (see, for example, Hatfield (2003), p. 162), bodies could count as eminent causes of sensory ideas. I thank Martha Bolton for pointing out this possible objection to me. Second, it is questionable whether possessing the property of extension is sufficient for Descartes to place body on a lower level on the ontological scale given that his ontological hierarchy seems to imply only a classification of things into infinite substances, finite substances and modes of those substances.

[32] See Schmaltz (1992), p. 40 and p. 48.

in arguing that the Objective Reality Principle *allows* (rather than precludes) the causal action of bodies on minds.[33] First, Schmaltz points out that this *must* be the case because Descartes, in Meditation Six, employs the objective reality principle to prove that bodies exist as long as they are the causes of our sensory ideas:

> Indeed in Meditation VI [Descartes] appealed explicitly to the Objective Reality Principle in support of [the claim that bodies cause sensory ideas]. He argues there that the cause of sensory ideas must formally or eminently contain what is contained objectively in these ideas. After affirming that it is inconsistent with the veracity of God that the cause of these ideas eminently contain this objective reality, Descartes concludes that bodies must cause the ideas [. . .]. He simply *assumes* that bodies formally contain what is contained objectively in sensory ideas.[34]

Second, and more importantly, Schmaltz *explains why* Descartes is entitled to make the assumption that bodies formally contain what is contained objectively in sensory ideas. He begins by defending the claim that ideas of secondary qualities, like all ideas, have both formal and objective reality.[35] Their formal reality consists in their being mental acts with a certain phenomenal content. And in defense of the controversial claim that ideas of secondary qualities have objective reality, Schmaltz quotes the passage in Meditation Three where Descartes writes that sensory ideas, like all ideas, are "as it were the images of things" (CSM II 25; AT VII 37); and the passage in Meditation Six where Descartes claims that there is a link between the various sensations of heat, colour and so on and *some qualities in bodies*:

> [. . .] from the fact that I perceive by my senses a great variety of colors, sounds, smells and tastes, as well as differences in heat, hardness and the like, I am

[33] Ibid., p. 44. Janet Broughton, Daisie Radner and, more recently, Geoffrey Gorham (among others) have defended the view that the similarity condition on causation precludes body-to-mind causation. See Broughton (1986), Gorham (2002) and Radner (1971). Their reasoning is (roughly) as follows. The causal principle requires that bodies contain properties that are the same as the properties contained objectively in the sensory ideas; but Descartes holds that bodies are only to be characterized in terms of extension, size and figure; so bodies do not literally contain, for example, the colors that we experience. So, bodies cannot *cause* our sensations of color. They can, at best, occasion them.

[34] Schmaltz (1992), p. 45, emphasis added.

[35] Ibid., p. 43, p. 45 and p. 48.

correct in inferring that the bodies which are the sources of these various sensory perceptions possess differences corresponding to them, though not resembling them. (CSM II 56; AT VII 81)

But in order to follow Schmaltz's argument completely, it is necessary to dwell a little longer on what exactly are the qualities of bodies that, according to Schmaltz, are contained objectively in ideas of sense. The claim in the above passage that ideas of sense are linked to properties of bodies *without resembling them*; and Schmaltz's reference to Descartes' claim in Meditation Six that the objective reality of sensory ideas corresponds only to the properties of bodies that we clearly and distinctly understand (CSM II 55; AT VII 80), indicate that the properties of bodies sensory ideas contain objectively (or represent) are the primary qualities of bodies. So, according to Schmaltz, Descartes' view is that sensory ideas have objective reality insofar as they direct the mind towards objects in space or represent bodies as having the properties of extension, shape and size.[36]

And once we distinguish between the formal and objective reality of ideas this way, we can argue that bodies are proper causes of our sensory ideas as follows. Although bodies cannot be the causes of the ideas as modes of awareness (since there is nothing in bodies that is the same as the phenomenological aspect of experience) bodies can be the causes of the objective reality of ideas (since bodies contain *the same properties* of extension and shape that are contained objectively in the ideas). Bodies are, then, only partial formal causes of sensory ideas. *They are the formal causes of the objective reality (or representational content) of sensory ideas.* The mind is the formal cause of their phenomenal content.[37] Here's how Schmaltz summarizes his view:

[sensory ideas] objectively contain qualities of bodies in the sense that these ideas can *direct* the mind to certain bodily qualities in virtue of the fact that

[36] This reading is further confirmed by the following passage in Schmaltz (1992): "Bodies formally contain what is in the sensory ideas objectively [...] in the sense that they possess the qualities to which these ideas direct the mind. Admittedly, this reading stretches thin Descartes' claim in the Second Replies that properties contained objectively in ideas are contained formally in bodies only when they exist outside of mind in a way that is 'such as [...] we perceive them' (AT VII 161; CSM II 114) But I take Descartes' own remarks concerning confused and obscure sensory ideas to suggest a rather thin notion of 'being as such' these ideas reveal" (Schmaltz (1992), pp. 46–47).

[37] Ibid., p. 48.

variations in ideas are linked to variations in these qualities. One obvious way in which the relevant sort of link could be established is by means of a causal connection between ideas and bodies. *The fact that ideas possess objective reality that directs the mind to bodily qualities indicates that they are linked to such qualities, and the fact that they are linked to these qualities indicates that they are caused by (or in Descartes' words), come from bodies.*[38]

So, on the one hand, sensory ideas have objective reality (i.e., they are directed towards extended bodies) because they are caused by extended bodies. On the other hand, what underwrites the causal connection between extended bodies and sensory ideas (as the causal principle implies) is the *similarity* between the cause and *how* the cause is *represented* (that is, the similarity between the extended body and the representation of the cause *as an extended body*). This is how Schmaltz argues for a causal account of the representationality of Cartesian sensations. However, in the following section, I will explain why this argument creates more problems than it solves for a supporter of a causal account of sensory representation.[39]

Although Schmaltz does not centre his discussion of Cartesian sensations around the solution of the puzzle of misrepresentation, his explanation of misrepresentation is similar to Wilson's. What allows Descartes to characterize sensory ideas as systematic "representations of their objects *as other than* they are" is the fact that sensory ideas (referentially) represent their right objects in virtue of a causal connection with them. So, ideas referentially represent their true objects independently of how they present them to the mind. In fact, Schmaltz writes, although sensory ideas "represent the qualities of bodies in [a] broad sense" (and here "represent the qualities of bodies" must be taken *de re*), "the mind cannot know simply by introspection which qualities these ideas represent: that is why Descartes called such ideas confused and obscure."[40] Accordingly, sensory ideas misrepresent because what

[38] Ibid., p. 47, emphasis added.

[39] One could object that Schmaltz's point is precisely to *deny* that bodies cause sensory ideas in virtue of a relation of similarity. But this cannot be the case. Although Schmaltz does not phrase the argument the way I did, the argument summarized above (*contra* the objection) must be the argument he has in mind. This is confirmed by the dialectic of the article. Schmaltz is defending the view that bodies are causes of sensory ideas by appealing to what he calls "the formal containment principle" and he describes this principle as implying a similarity condition even when it is applied to sensory ideas. See Schmaltz (1992), pp. 46–47.

[40] Ibid., p. 46.

they presentationally represent to the mind is different from what the ideas referentially represent. But unlike Wilson, Schmaltz does not distinguish between a presentational and referential sense of representation along the lines of a two-factor theory. He distinguishes the *phenomenal* content from the *representational* content of ideas. But since he does not distinguish between a referential and presentational sense of *representation* and he wants to explain the *representationality* of sensation in terms of a causal connection, I take him to be saying that the causal connection explains not only why the idea of *n* refers to *ns* (since it is caused by *ns* in the right why) but also why it says of *ns that they are ns* (that is, why it presents its object *as n*).[41] Keeping this in mind will be relevant for evaluating the prospects of Schmaltz's account to solve the puzzle of misrepresentation.[42]

3.5 SCHMALTZ'S CA AND PROBLEMS (A)–(D)

In this section, I will claim that Schmaltz's account offers no better solution than Wilson's to problems (b) and (d), but that it has the resources for providing (at least, *prima facie*) an answer to problems (c), and consequently, (a). I will contend, however, that the solution to problem (c) unwillingly reintroduces an internalist element into Descartes' account of the representationality of sensation and, hence, ends up undermining the very account it is supposed to defend.

[41] That is, unlike Wilson, Schmaltz is really following the guidelines of a causal theory of content as outlined by Fodor in the passage in section 3.3.2 above.

[42] Notice that Wilson and Schmaltz (see also Hoffman (1996)) agree that the causal connection holds between the mind and bodies or particular configurations of matter. Recently, this view has been criticized by Thomas Vinci. Vinci argues that the causes of ideas of bodies are the corporeal images in the brain rather than bodies. See Vinci (2008). Accordingly, he also maintains that the direct objects of our sensory ideas are the corporeal images in the brain and that the sensory representation of particular objects like the sun is the result of a judgment. Although intriguing, I disagree with Vinci mainly on textual grounds. For example, I take Descartes to deny in the *Optics* that the mind looks at images in the brain (CSM I 167; AT VI 130) and I take the proof of the existence of bodies in Meditation Six to be based on the claim that sensory ideas are caused by bodies. I do not discuss Vinci's position in full in this context because his account deals primarily with sensory ideas such as the ideas of the sun rather than with ideas of secondary qualities.

I will discuss problems (a)–(d) in the order that is most conducive to deliver the punch line of this section. I will start with problem (b), that is, the problem of explaining sensory misrepresentation within the framework of CA. As we saw in 3.4 above, Schmaltz, along the lines of a genuine causal theory of content, explains why ideas both present and refer to their objects in virtue of a causal connection. The causal connection explains why the idea of red says *of* red *that it is red.* However, Schmaltz's account, even more clearly than Wilson's, is vulnerable to the objection that a causal theory cannot explain misrepresentation. According to a causal theory, ideas represent what causes them. Consequently, since what causes the idea of red is a mode of *res extensa* either the idea of red says *of* red that *it is a mode of res extensa* or if it says *of* red that *it is something other than a mode of res extensa,* then it is not the idea of red (see 3.3.2 above).

Schmaltz would probably dismiss this objection and claim instead that one can easily explain why the idea of red can say *of* red that it is *something other than a mode of res extensa* as follows. The idea of red does not present red as a mode of *res extensa* because sensory ideas are confused and, so, the subject cannot tell from mere introspection of the content of the ideas *what* object they actually represent. But the above objection cannot be dismissed so quickly. Notice that the claim that, in the case of sensory ideas, the right object of the idea (i.e., a mode of *res extensa*) causes an obscure and confused representation of itself amounts to sheer contradiction. For the implication is that, on the one hand, the causal connection with the right object determines *what* the idea represents; but on the other hand, the same causal connection with the right object does *not* determine what the idea represents (since the representation is obscure). But let's assume that there is no contradiction here, for argument's sake. And let's assume that the view is that the true object of the idea (i.e., a mode of *res extensa*) causes in us the *confused representation of itself* (i.e., the representation of a mode of *res extensa* as resembling the sensation). The following question would still need answering: how can a causal theory (according to which the idea presents the property whose instances cause it) explain the fact that the (right) object of the idea causes a *confused* representation of itself in the mind? How does it happen that the causal impact of bodies on the mind produces a confused representation of bodies? Schmaltz does not address this question.

As far as I know, only Paul Hoffman – who has defended a causal account of Cartesian sensations which is similar in many respects to Schmaltz's – has acknowledged this problem and provided a possible answer to the above question.[43] Hoffman points out that the Scholastics had similar difficulties in explaining sensory misrepresentations. According to the Scholastic theory of cognition "a sensory idea cannot be caused by something other than what it presentationally represents because (i) it presentationally represents what exists objectively in the soul and (ii) what exists objectively in the soul is the same as what *produces* it."[44] But Hoffman points out that Aquinas and Ruvio offered explanations of cases of misrepresentation even on this model of cognition. In the case of proper sensibles (such as color, sound and so on), according to Aquinas and Ruvio, if the form of sweetness (for example) is received improperly by the soul due to a defect in the sense organ the subject may experience bitterness. Accordingly, the form of sweetness can exist objectively in the soul while appearing other than it actually is.[45] Likewise, Hoffman suggests, according to Descartes, modes of *res extensa* can exist objectively in the mind although they appear other than they actually are. As he puts it, "perhaps Descartes would be willing [...] to assert [...] that modes of bodies existing objectively in our sensations are sufficiently obscure that they appear as colors."[46] I take it that the suggestion is that, according to Descartes, the representation of modes of *res extensa* is received improperly by the mind due to some defect of the sense organs and this explains why the mind experiences modes of *res extensa* (confusedly) as similar to the sensation.

But this proposed answer to the above question raises two difficulties. First, it implies more explicitly than in Schmaltz's case (as we shall see below) the problematic claim that the representation of the properties of bodies for Descartes comes from bodies themselves. I will discuss this implication below. Second, it is questionable whether we can explain the notion of confused representation by appealing to the *defectiveness* of

[43] See Hoffman (1996).

[44] Ibid., p. 366, emphasis added.

[45] Ibid., p. 367: "[...] in the [...] case of the proper sensibles, [according to Aquinas] we can have a false cognition only if the sense organ is defective and the sensible is not received properly. So [Aquinas] explains that sweet things seem bitter to sick people because of the corruption of the tongue."

[46] Ibid., p. 378. See also: "[According to Descartes], the idea of cold is a mode of extension existing in our mind so obscurely that it appears as cold" (Ibid., p. 379).

the sense organs in Descartes' case. Since in the case of secondary qualities, according to Descartes, misrepresentation is the norm, we ought to conclude that the sense organs are defective in the perception of color and, so, in normal circumstances. But this is not Descartes' view.[47] I conclude that Hoffman does not provide a satisfactory answer to the above question, which then still remains unanswered. And, so, CA (in all its variations) fails to provide a satisfactory explanation of the phenomenon of misrepresentation.

Schmaltz has recently conceded that the *qua*-problem (i.e., problem (d) above) indicates that a causal link alone is not sufficient to fix the object of sensory ideas and has suggested that the causal account needs to be complemented with a teleofunctional account along the lines of Simmons (1999).[48] I will discuss teleofunctional accounts in Chapter 4 below. For the time being, let me just point out that, assuming the task of a theory of content consists precisely in explaining why ideas represent what they do, a causal theory that needs another theory of content to specify why ideas represent what they do hardly counts as a *causal* theory of content.

Problem (c) raises the question of whether effects can be *inherent* representations of their causes. Schmaltz's causal account, at least *prima facie*, fares better than Wilson's in countering this objection since it seems to have the resources for explaining why a sensory idea is an inherent representation of its cause. Effects of bodies on minds are inherent representations of their causes in virtue of a relation of *similarity* between cause and effect. The effect is a representation of the cause because the former resembles the latter. As Schmaltz puts it:

> My suggestion is that Descartes sometimes thought that even *though bodily qualities are not "entirely such as" sensory ideas reveal them to be*, still the *qualities are contained objectively in these ideas* [. . .] in the sense that the ideas possess *something* that enables the mind to be directed to these qualities.[49]

Schmaltz claims here that although sensory ideas are not accurate representations of the properties of bodies, the ideas objectively contain

[47] See for example, Descartes' discussion of the case of dropsy in Meditation Six.

[48] This concession does not appear in print since it represents a recent development of Schmaltz's views. Schmaltz informed me about this recent development in a private exchange.

[49] Schmaltz (1992), p. 47, my emphasis.

these properties and it is *in virtue of* this objective containment that they are directed towards bodies. That is, the *something* that directs the ideas towards bodies is the *similarity* between the properties of bodies (obscurely) represented in the idea and the actual properties of bodies. Consequently, there is no need of mediating intentions in order to explain why an idea becomes a representation of its cause and so problems (c) (and (a)) are solved.[50] Sensory represent bodies because they are semi-correct "images" of them.

However, Schmaltz's solution to this problem is not satisfactory either in light of Descartes' own philosophy or on theoretical grounds. *First*, causal accounts are usually invoked to explain mental representation as opposed to other accounts that explain it in virtue of *a relation of similarity or resemblance*. Aside from the fact that Wilson introduces causal accounts to defy the view that resemblance is a necessary condition for representation, Descartes himself clearly intended his causal story of the origin of sensation (whatever it amounts to) to be a criticism of the Scholastic resemblance theory of perception.[51] And, so, Schmaltz's reintroduction of the notions of similarity and resemblance in order to provide a *causal* account of the representationality of sensation is, at least, puzzling.

One could object that we should keep the notions of resemblance and similarity separate. The notion of similarity is a metaphysical condition on body-to-mind causation and, as such, it has to be kept distinct from resemblance as a condition for representation. But there are at least two

[50] For a similar account of the representationality of sensation see Hoffman (1996), pp. 375–376.

[51] For example, Descartes writes in the *Optics*: "We must take care not to assume – as our philosophers commonly do – that in order to have sensory perceptions the soul must contemplate certain images transmitted by objects to the brain; or at any rate we must conceive the nature of these images in an entirely different manner from that of the philosophers. For since their conception of the images is confined to the requirement that they should resemble the objects they represent, the philosophers cannot possibly show us how the images can be formed by the objects, or how they can be received by the external sense organs and transmitted by the nerves to the brain" (CSM I 165; AT VI 112). And after this passage, Descartes continues: "[…] we must not think that it is by means of its resemblance [to the objects from which it proceeds] that the picture causes our sensory perception of these objects […]. Instead we must hold that it is the movements composing this picture which, acting directly upon our soul in so far as it is united to our body, are ordained by nature to make it have such sensations. […] [T]here need be no resemblance between the ideas which the soul conceives and the movements which cause these ideas" (CSM I 167; AT VI 130–131).

problems with this objection. First of all, it is not clear what kind of similarity there is between the bodily properties of extension and the *representation* of these properties. Second, the aim of a causal theory is to explain why ideas of sense represent properties of bodies in the first place. This is what Schmaltz wants to account for. He intends to explain not only body-to-mind causation but also the *representationality* of sensation in virtue of a causal connection. And although the similarity condition certainly allows us to explain body-to-mind causation, it still does not answer the question of *why* sensory ideas *happen to contain objectively the properties of bodies* in virtue of whose similarity bodies are said to cause these ideas. So, as long as we think of similarity as a metaphysical condition, we may have an explanation of why the causal action of bodies on mind is permitted but no explanation of *why* ideas *represent* their causes (*viz.*, bodies) in virtue of a similarity relation. This last remark takes me to the second and third difficulties I want to raise.

Second, Schmaltz's explanation of the representationality of sensations is suspiciously circular. Sensory ideas are said to be directed towards (i.e., represent) bodies because they are caused by them. However, bodies are said to be able to cause these ideas *because* the properties of bodies are similar to the representational content of the ideas. But, then, the representational content of the idea must be available before, and independently of, a causal explanation (on pain of circularity). In conclusion, it must be the very *nature* of the representational content of sensory ideas that allows the causal explanation of their representational content rather than being the causal connection that explains the nature of the representational content of the ideas.[52]

In summary, either Schmaltz's account only aims at laying out the necessary metaphysical conditions for body-to-mind causation and then leaves the question of the representationality of sensory ideas unanswered; or it is (as I think it is) a causal account of the representationality

[52] As Thomas Vinci has pointed out to me, this conclusion can be also expressed in a slightly different way as a general problem for a causal theory. According to a causal theory an idea represents its (correct) object if and only if it is caused by it in the right way. But notice that knowing the "correct" object is necessary to spell out what it means for an idea to be caused in the right way. And this creates a circularity for "being caused in the right way" is supposed to *explain what* the idea represents. Hence, the idea's representation of its correct object must be independent of (and prior to) the "right" causal connection with the environment.

of sensations, but then it ends up presupposing, rather than providing, an account of the representational content of sensory ideas. Notice that this second point follows from what I said above *unless* one is prepared to defend the claim that, for Descartes, causal interaction is sufficient to explain the representationality of sensation because bodies, so to speak, imprint their own properties on the mind. Consideration of this point will take me to the third difficulty I want to raise. But first I want to consider two possible objections to my charge of circularity.

It could be objected that the main idea of causal theories is precisely that we can introspect the representational content of the idea *without* knowing what causes it since these two notions are distinct. Consequently, the accusation of circularity would be undermined.[53] However, this is not what Schmaltz claims. Schmaltz claims that – no matter how confused – sensory ideas objectively contain the primary qualities of bodies; and that it is this objective containment that (together with the similarity between the represented and actual properties of bodies) *tells us* what the objects/causes of the ideas are and *allows* (metaphysically speaking) the causal interaction. It follows, then, that we *cannot* introspect the representational content of the idea *without* knowing what causes it, and so, the threat of circularity is reinstated.

One could also object that to claim that Schmaltz's explanation of the representationality of sensation is circular is as absurd as to claim the following: "the explanation of why the motion of a first billiard ball causes motion in a second billiard ball in virtue of a similarity relation is circular because one would need to know about the motion of the second ball first."[54] However, notice that the analogy between the two explanations is faulty. In the case of the billiard balls, what needs to be explained is why the first ball can explain the *occurrence* of the motion in the second ball. And, so, it is unproblematic to presuppose knowledge of the motion of the second ball. But in Schmaltz's case, the causal connection needs to explain the *representational content* of the sensation rather than its *occurrence* and, so, it does not seem as unproblematic to presuppose knowledge of the representational content.

Third, (and this third point reinforces the second one and justifies the first one), Schmaltz claims that sensory ideas represent the primary qual-

[53] Thanks to Thomas Vinci for pointing out this possible objection.
[54] I owe this objection to Desmond Hogan.

ities of bodies because they are caused by them in the right way. But short of assuming that bodies actually *imprint* the representation of these properties on the mind, no explanation is provided of how the causal connection *alone* can succeed in explaining why ideas end up *representing* these properties. But Descartes certainly did not think either that these qualities of bodies are passively received by the mind or that their representation comes from the objects themselves.[55] On the contrary, the ideas of body and extension, figure, number and so on are innate to the mind.[56]

Because of the above difficulties, *contra* Schmaltz, there cannot be a purely causal explanation of the *representationality* of Cartesian sensations. Schmaltz wants to say that there is *something* in ideas that directs them towards bodies. It is also clear that this something is the representation of the primary qualities of bodies. However, as I argued above, *there cannot be a causal explanation of how this "something" that directs sensory ideas towards bodies ends up being in the mind.* The alternative (suggested, in passing, in the discussion of the third difficulty above) is that *the directionality comes from the mind itself* – in particular from the innate ideas of body and extension which are implicitly employed in the sensory representation of reality.[57] I conclude that Schmaltz's very solution to problem (c) – that is, his attempt to spell out the nature of the causal relation between bodies and ideas in terms of similarity – *unwillingly* highlights the necessity of reintroducing an internalist element in Descartes' account of sensory representation and, so, ends up undermining the very account it is supposed to support. The solution to problem (c) (and (a)) is then debunked, and the internalist reading of the objective reality of ideas of Chapter 1 is (somewhat) vindicated.

CONCLUSION

Problems (a)–(d) and the self-defeating character of Schmaltz's causal account indicate not only that Descartes did not hold a purely causal theory of the representationality of sensations but also that an internalist

[55] See CSM I 172; AT VI 140–141; CSM I 304; AT VIIIB 359 and CSM II 21; AT VII 31.

[56] CSM II 21; AT VII 31; CSMK 226–227; AT III 691; CSM II 44; AT VII 63–64.

[57] I will develop, and defend, this claim in Chapter 5.

element must be taken into consideration in accounting even for Descartes' views on sensory representation. Our discussion suggests that Descartes' view on the role of the causal connection between the mind and bodies was more complex than causal accounts may want (or afford) to concede. Descartes' view, as it emerges from the above discussion, seems to be along the following lines: sensory ideas do not represent their objects simply in virtue of being caused by them in the right way. Rather, ideas of bodies are caused by bodies in the right way *because* they (i.e., the ideas) *already* represent them *as* bodies. In other words, the mind could not output the representation *of* bodies as a result of a causal link with the environment unless it already conceived the cause *as a* body.

Since CA cannot explain the phenomenon of sensory misrepresentation and Schmaltz's version of CA reveals the necessity of complementing the causal story with an internalist one, I conclude that the prospects of solving the exegetical issue of sensory misrepresentation lie in understanding the interplay between an internalist and a causal element in Descartes' account of sensory representation. I will develop and defend this reading of Descartes in detail in Chapter 5 below. But before I do that I want to discuss a different externalist account of Cartesian sensations, *viz.*, a teleofunctional one.

4

Externalist Solutions: Teleofunctional Accounts

Many scholars have suggested that, according to Descartes, the intellect has the cognitive task of discovering the true nature of reality whereas sensations have the bio-functional task of securing "the preservation of the healthy man" (CSM II 60; AT VII 87).[1] Alison Simmons has developed this reading of Descartes into an externalist interpretation of the representational content of sensations.[2] Rethinking the role of the senses this way, claims Simmons, suggests that, according to Descartes, "sensations represent things in the corporeal world [. . .] in virtue of the role they play in enabling us to interact with the environment in a self-preserving way."[3] I will call this account "teleofunctional" (TA).

TA offers an externalist explanation of the representationality of Cartesian sensations that builds on, but differs from, CA. The main similarities and differences between CA and TA can be put succinctly as follows. According to both accounts, sensations represent things in the corporeal world in virtue of being locked into a causal connection with the environment. However, according to TA, the content-determining causal connections are selected by the biological function of the senses. This divergence results in different conclusions about the properties of bodies that cause and, hence, are represented by, sensations. According to TA, sensations are caused by and, hence, represent, ecological properties of

[1] See, for example, Gueroult (1985), pp. 97–176; Rodis-Lewis (1990), chapters one and two; MacKenzie (1990); Rorty (1986); Hatfield (1998) and (2003); and Alanen (1994) and (2003).

[2] See Simmons (1999). According to Alison Simmons, we should take the passages where Descartes talks about the biological role of the senses "as containing [...] rich materials for a new account of the nature of sensory representation" (Simmons (1999), p. 355).

[3] Ibid., p. 357.

bodies since the representation of these properties is what allows sensations to fulfill their biological function. According to CA, instead, sensations are caused by, and represent, the mathematical and geometrical properties of bodies (or modes of *res extensa*).

Simmons contends that TA is superior to CA because it is textually more accurate and because it solves (some of) CA's main difficulties. In particular, one of the main advantages of TA would consist in dissolving the exegetical problem that motivates CA, i.e., the problem of sensory misrepresentation. According to Simmons, since the role of the senses consists in preserving the health of the mind–body union, sensations represent the corporeal world not as-it-is-in-itself but as-it-is-in-relation-to-the-mind–body-union; and, as long as they do that successfully, they are "materially true," that is, they are correct representations of their objects.[4]

In this chapter, I argue that, despite its *prima facie* attractiveness, TA cannot be attributed to Descartes because it lacks textual support, it introduces more theoretical problems than it solves, and it is not superior to (but rather inherits some of the problems of) CA. Since Simmons has offered the most extensive defense of this new way of understanding the representationality of Cartesian sensations, I make Simmons (1999) the primary critical target of this chapter.[5] I begin by presenting Simmons' TA and its alleged advantages (4.1). Then, I will argue that TA and its proposed solution to the puzzle of misrepresentation raise several theoretical problems (4.2, 4.3.1, 4.3.2); and that, even if we were prepared to disregard these problems, TA does not have the advantage of solving the problem of misrepresentation that it is advertised as having (4.2.1, 4.3.3). I conclude by providing an alternative reading of the teleological jargon of Meditation Six that shows that this text (*contra* Simmons' claim) does not in any straightforward way support TA.

4.1 A TELEOFUNCTIONAL ACCOUNT (TA)

According to Simmons, Descartes, in Meditation Six, denies that the intellect and the senses are joined in the common cognitive task of

[4] See Simmons (1999), pp. 353–356. This will become clearer in section 4.1 below.

[5] For a teleofunctional interpretation of Descartes' view on the passions that is inspired by Simmons (1999) and Simmons (2001), see Greenberg (2007).

discerning the true nature of reality. Rather, Descartes claims that the senses have "the biological function [. . .] to guide our [. . .] self-preserving interaction with bodies in local environment [and, hence] have their own job to do."[6] The biological function of the senses, argues Simmons, suggests that Descartes tendered a teleofunctional account of sensory representation, according to which sensations "represent things *in the corporeal world* [. . .] not simply in virtue of being caused in the right way by those things, but *in virtue of* the role they play in enabling us to interact with the environment in a self-preserving way."[7] Accordingly, sensations represent primarily *ecological properties* of bodies rather than their mathematical and geometrical properties. Ecological properties, writes Simmons, describe to the mind "what bodies (its own included) are like, not in themselves as conceived by the Cartesian physicist but relative to its own body's well-being."[8] Ecological properties of bodies, then, are defined by an element of indexicality: where is this body relative to *my* body? Will this body pose a threat to *me*? And examples of these properties are *bodily damage, bodily health* and *surface differences.*[9]

The strongest support for TA is found in Meditation Six. For example, after having remarked that God has instituted the one-to-one relation between brain states and sensations that is "most frequently conducive to the preservation of the healthy man," Descartes explains:

> [W]hen the nerves in the foot are set in motion in a violent and unusual manner, this motion, by way of the spinal cord, reaches the inner parts of the brain, and there gives the mind its signal for having a certain sensation, namely the sensation of a pain as occurring in the foot. This stimulates the mind to do its best to get rid of the cause of the pain, which it takes to be harmful to the foot. It is true that God could have made the nature of man such that this particular motion in the brain indicated something else to the mind; it might, for example, have made the mind aware of the actual motions occurring [. . .] in the foot [. . .]. But there is nothing else which would have been so conducive to the continued well-being of the body. (CSM II 60–61; AT VII 88)

[6] Simmons (1999), p. 355.
[7] Ibid., p. 357. Emphasis added.
[8] Ibid., p. 355.
[9] "Pains represent bodily damage, tickles represent bodily health [. . .] color sensations represent surface differences" (Ibid., p. 356).

According to Simmons, the above passage suggests that the *biological function* of the sensation of pain as occurring in the foot (i.e., that of doing something to get rid of the pain) explains both (a) why the sensation represents its distal cause (i.e., a real injury in the foot) rather than any other of the more proximate causes (i.e., the pineal gland state or some motions in the medium between the distal cause and the sensation); and (b) why it *phenomenally* represents the cause as *pain* rather than as what the cause is really like.[10] In short, the biological function of sensation explains why sensations represent *what* they do (their referential content) and why they represent it *the way* they do (their presentational content). Notice that the presentational content of sensation would contain not only the presentation of the object that causes the sensation (i.e., some ecological property) but also the non-descriptive, or phenomenal, presentation of it.

I want to pause here and discuss (a) above at more length. Notice that (a) implies that, according to TA, the causal connection between a sensation and its right cause is subordinate to the biological role of sensation. Accordingly, Cartesian sensations are caused by (and, hence, represent) their "right" objects in virtue of their role of enabling us to navigate the environment in a self-preserving way. So, the fact that a representational state S veridically represents its object (or is caused by its right object) is explained in terms of the biological function of S. When Descartes writes that the sensation of pain-as-if-in-the-foot represents an injury in the foot because it is caused by it in normal circumstances, we should define these normal circumstances as those that promote the well-being of the mind–body union. Consequently, the senses' *function* of preserving the health of the man explains why it is an injury in the foot that *causes* the sensation of pain-as-if-in-the-foot and, hence, why sensations are by and large veridical.

Moreover, according to Simmons, Descartes must be committed to (a) if we want to provide an externalist explanation of his account of sensory representation that avoids the pitfalls of CA. As we saw in 3.3.4 above, CA is threatened by what is known as the "*qua* problem." The problem is that since, according to CA, a representational state S

[10] Simmons (1999), p. 357. See also Simmons (2001), p. 56.

represents what causes it and S is caused by any number of different causes, a causal account of what S represents is bound to fail. Suppose the representational state S is the sensation of pain as if in the foot. Its cause is not only its distal cause (i.e., an actual injury in the foot) but also any other cause in the chain that goes from the distal cause to the sensation – for instance, a pineal gland state. How can a causal theory explain why S represents its distal cause rather than any other cause? Simmons describes this problem as the failure of a causal theory of isolating "in a principled way the distal cause *as* the proper *res repraesentata* of a sensation."[11] TA's advantage consists in providing Descartes with this principled reason. "As [Descartes] says," writes Simmons, "what we most need to know *about* to survive is the usual distal cause. We thus have reason to affirm what phenomenologically seems to be the case, e.g., that color sensations represent to us the surfaces of distal bodies."[12] In other words, the biological function explains why the reference-fixing causal connection is the one with the distal cause and, hence, why the mind *outputs* the representation of an external body (or distal cause) as opposed to the representation of a pineal gland state (even if the sensation is caused by the external body-or-pineal gland state). So, again, TA is in a better position than CA to account for why sensations are, by and large, veridical. The biological functions of the senses explains why color sensations are caused by, and hence represent, the surfaces of actually existing bodies and why the sensation of pain-as-if-in-the-foot is caused by, and hence represents, a real injury in the foot.

To summarize, TA consists of two basic claims: (1) sensations represent *different* objects than the intellect, *viz.*, the *ecological* properties of the corporeal world; and (2) sensations represent ecological properties *in virtue of* their biological function. Because of (1) and (2), argues Simmons, sensations "represent the corporeal world [. . .] exactly as they ought to [and, so, are] materially true."[13] Since sensations represent the *ecological properties* of the corporeal world, they represent the corporeal world exactly as they ought to (*viz.*, in relation to the well-being of our body) and, so, they do not misrepresent it. So, one main advantage of TA

[11] Ibid., p. 353.
[12] Ibid., p. 361.
[13] Ibid., pp. 352–353.

over CA (and other theories) is that it dissolves the puzzle of sensory misrepresentation without denying that sensations are representational.

However, despite the fact that Descartes did claim that sensations help us navigate the surrounding environment, he did not hold TA. In sections 4.2 and 4.3, I will argue that the notion of ecological property and the functional accounts of representation and truth create more problems for Descartes than they allegedly solve (4.2, 4.3.1 and 4.3.2). Moreover, as we shall see, even if we ignore these problems, TA does not provide any straightforward solution to the puzzle of misrepresentation (4.2.1 and 4.3.3).

4.2 ECOLOGICAL PROPERTIES?

Simmons assumes a division of labor between the senses and the intellect. This division of labor implies that sensory and intellectual representations refer to "different things."[14] Sensations represent the ecological properties of bodies; intellections represent their geometrical properties. However, as Simmons herself acknowledges, ecological properties are *instantiated* in bodies as modes of *res extensa.*[15] In order to understand Simmons' view then, it becomes crucial to understand in what sense exactly, according to Simmons, ecological properties are *instantiated* in modifications of *res extensa.* However, no clarification of how to understand the relation of instantiation is provided. Is Descartes' view that ecological properties can be reduced to physical properties, or that ecological properties are realized in physical properties but are something over and above physical properties?[16] Simmons' interpretation requires Descartes to hold the latter. However, it is neither clear that Descartes held this view nor does Simmons make any attempt to defend it on Descartes' behalf.

But let's assume with Simmons that ecological properties are different from, yet instantiated in, modes of *res extensa.* And let's also assume with her that ecological properties are defined either (i) in relation to

[14] Simmons (1999), p. 356.

[15] Ibid., p. 356.

[16] Thanks to Martha Bolton for bringing this problem to my attention. When I say that ecological properties ought to be "over and above" physical properties I mean that they are different from the latter in the sense that they may be supervenient on, or emergent from, them.

well-being of the body[17]; or (ii) in relation to well-being of the mind–body union.[18] If Descartes' view is (i), then we have the following problem. Although it may be clear how bodily damage and health satisfy the definition of "ecological property" as a property defined in terms of the well-being of the body, it is not clear how surface differences do. In what sense are surface differences defined by the well-being of my body? Certainly, our ability to perceive differences among the surfaces of objects helps us navigate the environment successfully and, consequently, preserve the well-being of the body. However, the property of being a surface difference is not defined in terms of the well-being of the body like in the case of bodily health and damage. So, minimally, we would need some clarification of the difference between ecological properties such as "bodily health" and "being a surface difference." But Simmons provides none.

If Descartes' view is (ii) above, then sensations represent *properties-of-the-world-with-respect-to-the-survival-of-the-mind–body-union.* But are there any such properties, according to Descartes? If there are, they are distinct from the properties of the mind (as distinct from the body) and the properties of the body (as distinct from the mind). That is, (ii) seems to imply that ecological properties are properties of a third kind of substance, i.e., the mind–body union. But since it is not clear whether Descartes thought of the mind–body union as a third substance, a proponent of TA ought to either defend this interpretation of Descartes' view on the mind–body union or explain how (ii) above doesn't imply this reading of the mind–body union. But, again, no such clarification is in either Simmons (1999) or Simmons (2001).[19]

One may suggest that interpreting ecological properties as relational properties may explain Simmons' claim that ecological properties are

[17] Simmons (1999), p. 355.

[18] Simmons (2001), p. 58.

[19] Despite some passages where Descartes does seems to suggest that the mind and body are co-extensive and intermingle (for example, CSM II 56; AT VII 81; CSMK 226–229; AT III 690–695) it is not clear – and it is a matter of scholarly dispute – whether Descartes really held this view as opposed to the view that mind and body merely co-exist. On this see, for example, Wilson (1978), chapter six. I do not mean to suggest that Simmons explicitly endorses the former reading rather than the latter. On the contrary, she is very careful not to commit herself to either view of the mind–body union. However, this may be part of the problem. A full defense of her view seems to require a clarification of what the mind–body union is.

something over and above physical properties without committing Descartes to the problematic view that the mind–body union constitutes an independent third substance. A relational property is a property a thing has in virtue of being in relation to something else. One possible way of interpreting ecological properties as relational properties is to say that the former are properties of bodies as they appear to us (as conjunctions of mind and body) as opposed to as they are in themselves (i.e., modes of *res extensa*). So, for example, bodies' interaction with our body causes the perception of redness in virtue of the mind's connection with the human body. The property of redness as it appears to us, that is, the phenomenal red, is a mode of the mind–body union. The property of redness as a certain configuration of particles is a mode of *res extensa*. And this distinction would explain why ecological properties (such as the phenomenal red) are something over and above physical properties without postulating the existence of a third substance.[20]

However, this suggestion does not solve the problems raised above. First, one may agree that the phenomenal red is caused by a mode of *res extensa* (some particular configuration of particles) in virtue of the connection between the mind and the human body. In fact, according to Descartes, the sensation of red is nothing but the obscure and confused representation of the particular configuration of particles that caused the sensation. But notice that this is compatible with the view – held by CA – that sensations and the intellect represent the same thing just in two distinct ways. The senses represent modes of *res extensa* obscurely and confusedly; the intellect represents modes of *res extensa* clearly and distinctly. Second, the view that ecological properties are properties of bodies as they appear to us (or phenomenal properties) simply reduces to the view that, according to Descartes, modes of the mind (whether or not in connection with the human body) are irreducible to modes of body. Nobody would deny that this is Descartes' view but nobody would say that this amounts to a definition of an ecological property either. Besides, according to Simmons, ecological properties are still properties of *body* – even if defined in terms of the well-being of the mind–body union. So, the notion of phenomenal property is insufficient to explain the notion of ecological property.

[20] Thanks to Sean Greenberg for this suggestion.

But there is a different way of interpreting ecological properties as relational properties that avoids relating bodies to us and, hence, the above problems. It might be that ecological properties are properties *a thing has in virtue of the relation between its physical properties and the physical properties of our own body.* The property of being digestible is a function of the relation between the physical properties of the food and the physical properties of my body according to some physical laws. So, the suggestion is that ecological properties are *physical relational* properties. Accordingly, sensations would represent properties (for example, the property of being digestible) that are different from modes of *res extensa* even if ultimately ecological properties are modes of *res extensa.* This is the most charitable reading of ecological properties offered on behalf of Simmons and it might in the end be the best interpretation of what she *ought* to say. However, if this *were* what Simmons has in mind, she would have to defend this reading of ecological properties in the context of Descartes' metaphysics, especially in light of her additional claim that ecological properties ought to be defined in relation to the *well-being* of the mind–body union.[21] And would the above definition, for example, explain the sense in which surface differences count as ecological properties of bodies? So, at the very least, Simmons owes us some further explanation of ecological properties. Interpretation of their metaphysics should not be left to the reader.

4.2.1 Corollaries: TA and Misrepresentation

The lack of clarity regarding the ontological status of ecological properties has the unwelcome consequence of undermining TA's advertised advantage, *viz.*, that of dissolving the problem of misrepresentation. Simmons writes:

> The [. . .] advantage of [TA] is that it explains Descartes' response to the charge that God is a deceiver better than other interpretations. The charge [. . .] is that God is a deceiver since he has given us a sensory faculty that naturally gives rise to false judgments about the corporeal world. Descartes' response is [. . .] [that] the senses, [. . .] "report the *truth* more often than falsehood" (AT VII 89). The senses cannot report the truth without representing something. But they do not

[21] Simmons (1999), pp. 355–356.

report the truth about the nature or essence of the corporeal world. Once we get clear on the representational context of the senses, viz., the ecology of mind–body unions trying to survive in a world of other bodies, the truth of the senses stands out. The senses, Descartes is arguing, report the truth insofar as they represent to the mind the corporeal world's potential impact on the survival of its own body [...]. To put the point in more precise Cartesian terms, we should say that sensations are, with respect to bodily survival, *materially true.*[22]

Simmons' argumentative strategy is clear. The senses, differently from the intellect, have the job of representing the ecological properties of bodies (that is, the properties of the corporeal-world-as-it-is-with-respect-to-the-well-being of man); and insofar as sensations represent these properties, they represent bodies as they ought to and, so, they do not misrepresent them. They are *materially true.* So, the notion of ecological properties and its distinction from the geometrical and mathematical properties of bodies are essential to defend the claim that TA dissolves the problem of misrepresentation. However, as we saw in 4.2 above, it is unclear whether Descartes' metaphysics allows for either the notion of ecological property or its distinction from the essential properties of bodies. And this lack of clarity jeopardizes TA's advertised advantage.

If specifying the nature of the distinction between ecological and physical properties and physical properties is the source of all troubles, one may try to weaken the *distinction* between the things the senses and the intellect represent. Wouldn't representing the same objects in different ways be enough for Simmons' purposes (for example, to support her claim that sensations are materially true)?[23] However, weakening this distinction would undermine TA's capability of dissolving the problem of misrepresentation. As Simmons puts it, the "Cartesian distinction between intellect and senses [...] is not a distinction between a faculty that represents [...] well and one that represents poorly, but a distinction between faculties that represent *different things.*"[24] That is, the difference between what the senses and the intellect represent is not a difference at the presentational level but at the referential level. So, the distinction between *the things* represented by sensations and intellections is *central* to TA. Only if this distinction

[22] Simmons (1999), p. 363. Original emphasis.
[23] Thanks to Michael Della Rocca for this suggestion.
[24] Simmons (1999), p. 356, emphasis added.

can be sharply drawn, can we say that sensations are materially true and God is not a deceiver and, hence, that TA has advantages over CA. Once the distinction is gone, so are the advantages of TA.

However, Simmons herself at times acknowledges that sensations and intellections "represent different aspects of the same thing (in the corporeal world) to different ends."[25] This claim adds a further level of unclarity regarding the ontological status of ecological properties. Simmons acknowledges that sensations represent modes of *res extensa* indirectly by way of representing the ecological properties of the corporeal world and that these ecological properties are instantiated in modes of *res extensa.*[26] So, Simmons at times acknowledges that the senses and the intellect do represent the *same thing* (i.e. modes of *res extensa*). The claim that sensations represent *the same thing for different purposes* is not equivalent to the claim that they represent different things. However, notice that even if the senses and the intellect represent the same things for different purposes, the senses (insofar as they fall short of the clarity and distinctness of the intellect) *still misrepresent* their objects because they present them as other than they truly are and, hence, provide the potential for a mistaken judgment. And this is what Descartes means by calling sensations "materially false."

In conclusion, whether or not sensations are interpreted as representing ecological properties that are distinct from the geometrical and mathematical properties of bodies, TA's advertised advantage is in jeopardy. A sharp distinction between ecological and geometrical properties would dissolve the problem of misrepresentation but it is not obvious that Descartes' metaphysics supports this distinction. A weakened distinction between the two kinds of properties (as suggested by Descartes' claim that sensations represent modes of *res extensa* indirectly by way of representing ecological properties) would not be sufficient to establish that the senses provide a correct representation of reality.[27]

[25] Ibid., p. 356.

[26] Ibid., p. 356.

[27] Simmons claims that, on TA, misrepresentation is a much more limited phenomenon than on CA and illustrates this point as follows: "Compare a sensation of a ripe banana as yellow with a sensation of an unripe banana as yellow [...]. Both of these sensations represent banana surfaces as other than they corporeally are, but only the sensation of the ripe bananas as yellow conduces to self-preservation" (Ibid., p. 367, fn. 26). According to CA, both sensations are misrepresentations; according to TA only

4.3 TA AND THE VERIDICALITY OF SENSATIONS

As we saw in section 4.1 above, TA is supposed to explain the veridicality of sensation better than CA. The *biological function* of sensation explains the "correspondence" between the object presented to the mind (the presentational content) and the object the idea stands for (the referential content). For example, the biological function of the sensation of pain in the foot guarantees that the sensation is caused by (and, hence, represents) an injury in the foot. However, there are two (related) difficulties with this claim.

4.3.1 Teleology and Truth?

A teleological account of representation shifts the focus of attention on its securing the survival of the body rather than on its truth.[28] But then, on this view, it is possible to have a set of false beliefs that promote the well-being of the body as well as a set of true ones. And, so, there is the risk that truth may be severed from the biological function rather than being understood in its terms. We can imagine cognitive mechanisms that guarantee survival by systematically delivering false beliefs (as in the case when truths are too awful to bear). This criticism is intended as a *reductio* of Simmons' view. Once representation and truth are interpreted in terms of their function the possibility of cognitive mechanisms that systematically deliver false beliefs is left open and with it the possibility that truth may be severed from the biological function (*contra* the original hypothesis).[29]

one is. So, misrepresentation is a much more limited phenomenon on TA. This is an interesting point. However, saying that on TA misrepresentation is a much more limited phenomenon is not enough to support Simmons' claim that sensations are materially true, i.e., that they are not misrepresentations altogether.

[28] Simmons suggests a reinterpretation of the Cartesian notions of representation and misrepresentations in terms of function and malfunction, for example, in Simmons (1999), p. 367, fn. 26.

[29] Notice that the possibility of cognitive mechanisms delivering false beliefs is introduced by the very understanding of truth and representation in terms of their biological function rather than being the result of imagining radical skeptical scenarios.

One may object that this criticism presupposes a certain conception of *representation* as a mind–world relation and *truth* as correspondence between mental states and states of affair. Once these notions are revisited in terms of the conditions under which the biological function is fulfilled, the above criticism is dissolved. But *Descartes* didn't hold a functionalist theory of representational content and truth. Representationality is the property ideas have to cognitively present *the world* to us. Truth and representation, falsity and misrepresentation are explained *primarily* in terms of correspondence, or lack thereof, with reality (rather than in terms of function).[30] Understanding truth and representation in terms of their purposedness and ends is as foreign to Descartes' way of thinking as it was any explanation of natural phenomena in terms of their τέλος. And the strongest evidence for this is precisely Descartes' claim – *contra* Simmons' revision of Descartes – that sensory ideas are materially *false* ideas, i.e., ideas that are "referred to something other than that of which [they are] in fact the idea[s]" (CSM II 163; AT VII 233).

One could argue that the imagined scenario of a cognitive mechanism promoting survival and delivering false beliefs is *impossible*. Given that the function is selected in order to promote survival and false representations do not promote survival there is no risk of severing truth from the biological function. However, this response assumes that in order to select which sensations would better serve the function of securing survival we should already know what sensations represent (or whether they are true or false). But if this is the case, then a teleological account of sensations would presuppose an account of the representationality of sensations. This last remark takes us to the second difficulty I want to raise.

[30] For evidence that Descartes intended representation and truth primarily as a mind–world relation, see, for example, CSM II 26; AT VII 37; CSM II 54; AT VII 78; CSM II 193–201; AT VII 277–288; CSM II 249–252; AT VII 361–365. Amy Schmitter has pointed out to me (in a private exchange) that the passage in the Second Set of Replies where Descartes writes that "the perception whose truth we are so firmly convinced of may appear false to God or an angel" (CSM II 103; AT VII 145) may threaten my claim that Descartes endorsed a correspondence theory of truth. But it seems to me that, even if in a limited sense (with respect to the absolute point of view of God), truth for Descartes is still a matter of matching our clear and distinct ideas with reality. And this is all I need to say in order to contradict Simmons' suggestion that Descartes has a conception of truth according to which (roughly) a belief is true if it provides some benefits.

4.3.2 Presupposing an Account of Sensory Content

A teleological account of sensation *presupposes* rather than provides an account of sensory content. In order to say which conditions would normally make a sensation beneficial we would have to know what the sensation is about. So, specification of the normal circumstances in which a sensation is beneficial would presuppose *having* a theory of content and this defies the point of explaining content on the basis of what is beneficial to us. According to Simmons, the teleology of sensation determines the normal circumstances that fix the referent (or distal cause) of the sensory representation. So, for example, in normal circumstances the sensation of pain-as-if-in-the-foot is caused by a real damage in the foot because this is the most advantageous scenario for the survival of the mind–body union. However, in order to specify the normal circumstances under which a representational state would be beneficial to the mind–body union we would have to know first what the representational state is about. So, specification of the normal circumstances in which a sensation is beneficial would *presuppose* a theory of content.[31] *Mutatis mutandis*, selection of the normal circumstances in which a sensation is beneficial presupposes knowing that it is *veridical* and, so, the veridicality of sensation is not the result of the biological function (*contra* TA's claim).

This point highlights that TA (despite claims to the contrary) inherits some of the same difficulties as CA. Even if TA can answer the question of *why* the selected *res repraesentata* of sensation is the distal cause (as opposed to any of the proximate or intermediate causes), TA *fails as much as CA* to explain why sensations represent their distal causes in the first place. For, as I argued above, the fact that sensations represent external bodies *must* be presupposed by TA. And, so, although TA can answer the question of why the selected *res repraesentata* of sensations is an external body by saying that knowledge of external bodies is what we need to know most for survival, it still does not explain why the representation of external bodies is available to us in the first place. Consequently, TA fails as much as CA to fully solve the "qua-problem" because it fails to explain why sensations represent their causes *qua*

[31] On this point see Fodor (1993), chapter four.

external bodies. Specifying the biological function of sensation *presupposes* that sensations represent their causes *qua* external bodies, it does not explain it. This representational content must already be available in order for TA to specify the normal circumstances that promote survival.

4.3.3 Corollaries: TA and Misrepresentation

There are a few more reasons for questioning TA's advertised advantage in light of 4.3.1 and 4.3.2. First, as we saw in 4.3.2 above, if TA presupposes a theory of representational content, the solution of the puzzle of misrepresentation will depend on whatever theory of content is presupposed by TA.

Second, as we saw in 4.3.1 above, on TA, we can still have cases where the system is functioning well and yet sensations misrepresent their objects. Simmons suggests reinterpreting the notions of representation and misrepresentation in terms of function and malfunction. Accordingly, on TA, the sensory system is functioning well when the sensation of pain-as-if-in-the-foot is caused by an actual injury in the foot because these are the circumstances that promote the survival of the mind–body union. However, the sensory system is malfunctioning if the sensation-of-pain-as-if-in-the-foot is caused by some motions in the nerves other than in the foot (as in the case of amputees) because these circumstances will not necessarily promote a health-preserving behavior. However, Descartes points out that in cases when one has a sensation of pain-as-if-in-the-foot after one's foot has been amputated the system is *not malfunctioning*.[32] Yet we still want to say that, in this case, the sensation of pain in the foot misrepresents its object. In conclusion, even under TA, sensations are not always materially true (i.e., they may not represent the ecological properties that are supposed to represent) and consequently can give rise to erroneous judgments.

Third, if what the sensation represents is determined by its biological function; and the sensory system *functions equally well* both when the sensation of pain in the foot is caused by an injury in the foot and when the sensation of pain in the foot is caused by anything other than its distal cause (as in the case of the amputee); it follows that the notion of function is unable to fix which one among the various possible causes of

[32] See CSM II 58–59; AT VII 85.

a sensation is the correct one (*contra* Simmons' claim that this is a clear advantage of her TA over CA (see 4.1 above)).[33]

Fourth, there is another reason for doubting that TA solves the "qua-problem." Consider the sensation of pain as if in the foot. It is normally caused by its distal cause, that is, an injury in the foot. However, this sensation is also caused by intermediate causes such as movements in the nerves and pineal gland states. According to TA, the sensations of pain as if in the foot represents an injury in the foot rather than the other causes because the biological function of the sensation consists in promoting survival and only the causal connection between the sensation of pain as if in the foot and the injury in the foot guarantees survival. But in order for the sensation of pain as if in the foot to be causally connected with the distal cause it *must* also be connected with all the other intermediate causes. So, why doesn't the sensation of pain as if in the foot run the risk of representing a disjunction of causes even under TA?

In order to dismiss my second and third criticisms, one may reply that according to Descartes, the system is *indeed malfunctioning* when one has a sensation of pain-as-if-in-the-foot after one's foot has been amputated. In Meditation Six, one may continue, Descartes argues that (in the case of amputees) the system is still functioning well with respect to the body but *malfunctioning* with respect to the mind–body union as follows. Descartes distinguishes between (1) a sense of "nature" which takes into account the physical laws governing the human body seen as a "kind of machine" (CSM II 58; AT VII 84); and (2) a teleological sense of "nature" that takes into consideration the *purpose* of a certain physiological state (CSM II 58; AT VII 85).[34] Accordingly, when we say of someone suffering from dropsy that her nature is disordered we may be making two statements differing in truth-value depending on what

[33] One could invoke a distinction between ideal and non-ideal circumstances to distinguish between cases when the system functions well and cases when it doesn't. For example, one may say that a system is functioning well when, in ideal circumstances, it is attaining the goal of its function. In these ideal circumstances the sensation would indeed represent the distal cause. But it is not functioning well when, in non-ideal circumstances, the sensation represents the proximal cause. Notice, however, that although this distinction would rescue Simmons from the above criticism, it would still leave her with the problem of specifying the ideal circumstances in a way that does not already presuppose that the referent of the sensation is the distal cause (see 4.3.2 above).

[34] See Simmons (2001), pp. 58–59.

sense of "nature" we have in mind. If we are taking "nature" in sense (1) above, we are making a statement that does *not* correspond to matters of fact because no physical law is violated in the case of someone suffering from dropsy. But if we are taking "nature" in sense (2) above, so the objection goes, we are making a statement that corresponds to matters of fact. And so, in cases when one has a sensation of pain-as-if-in-the-foot after one's foot has been amputated the system is *indeed malfunctioning* (*contra* my above claim).

The successfulness of this rejoinder depends on how we read the passages in Meditation Six where Descartes distinguishes between these two senses of "nature" and on how we interpret his claim that the cases of dropsy and the amputee are "true errors of nature." The immediate context is the discussion of how to relieve God from the accusation of being a deceiver in the dropsy case and the like. We may say, Descartes suggests, that the nature of the patient suffering from dropsy is *disordered*. But that would not acquit God from deception since "a sick man is no less one of God's creatures than a healthy one" (CSM II 58; AT VII 84). The question arises of whether her nature is really "disordered." If we consider "nature" in sense (2) above we can say that the nature of the patient suffering from dropsy is disordered (CSM II 58; AT VII 85). However, comments Descartes, "nature" in this sense (i.e., the teleological sense) "*is simply a label which depends on my thought; it is quite extraneous to the things to which it is applied*" (CSM II 59; AT VII 85, emphasis added). So, if I am reading the text correctly, according to Descartes, when we are taking "nature" in the teleological sense we are not making a statement that *corresponds to matters of fact* when we say that the nature of someone suffering from dropsy is disordered.

One may rejoin that this reading doesn't take into consideration the passage that follows Descartes' distinction between a physical and teleological sense of nature:[35]

> When we say, then, with respect to the body suffering from dropsy that it has a disordered nature [. . .], the term "nature" is here used merely as an extraneous label. However, with respect to the composite [. . .] what is involved is not a mere label, but a true error of nature. (CSM II 59; AT VII 85)

[35] Simmons makes this remark in replying to a different objection to her view. See Simmons (2001).

According to Simmons, this passage clarifies in no uncertain terms "that the second sense of the term 'nature' (the teleological one) is a mere label *when attributed to the body* of the dropsy patient [. . .]. But [it] is not a mere label when attributed to the mind–body union."[36] In other words, according to Simmons, Descartes is making a further distinction within the teleological sense of nature (i.e., (2) above) as follows: (2)′ a teleological sense of nature with respect to the body; and (2)″ a teleological sense of nature with respect to the mind–body union. And only (2)′ would be a mere label that doesn't correspond to matter of fact.

I disagree with Simmons' interpretation of the text. When Descartes first introduces the teleological sense of nature and writes that nature in this sense is "a pure label that depends on my thought," he is *already* considering the teleological sense of nature *with respect to the mind–body union.* For, first, when Descartes introduces the teleological sense of nature he is contrasting it with the sense of "nature" that refers to the body as a machine with "no mind in it" (CSM II 58; AT VII 84). So, the contrast itself suggests that the teleological sense of nature regards "nature" as referring to the body united with the mind. Second, Descartes writes that the nature of the dropsy patient is disordered because "it [. . .] is deviating from its nature if the throat is dry at a time when drinking is not beneficial to its continued health" (CSM II 58; AT VII 85). The reference here to the state of health suggests that Descartes is talking about the body in conjunction with the mind. One may wonder whether it is only in reference with the mind (for example, as the house of the body) that the body can be said to be healthy or unhealthy.[37]

Finally, let's assume that Simmons is right and Descartes wants to say that the cases of dropsy and the amputee are true errors of nature. It still remains to be established in what sense they are "errors of nature." Simmons is assuming that they are errors of nature because they constitute a deviation from the proper purpose of sensations. But the text is not clear on this point. One could remark that the continuation of the last quoted passage ("It thus remains to inquire how it is that the goodness of God does not prevent nature, in this sense, from deceiving us" CSM II 59; AT VII 85) suggests that the errors of nature are

[36] See Simmons (2001), p. 58, original emphasis.
[37] Simmons only skirts this issue. Ibid., p. 55.

epistemic errors (at least insofar as God's deception is intended as the possibility that God may give us ideas that do not correspond to how things are). Accordingly, Descartes would be saying here that the cases of dropsy and the amputee are true errors of nature because they represent body as being in a state different from the state in which it actually is.[38] But then, if these are cases of epistemic errors, they cannot be used against my second and third criticisms above. Descartes would be treating them as cases of misrepresentations because they are false representations of their causes *rather than* because they deviate from the proper purpose of sensation. The system would be malfunctioning because it provides false representations rather than delivering false representation because it deviates from the proper purpose of sensations. But only in the latter case would Descartes' "true errors of nature" undermine my second and third criticisms. In sum, if a full defense of TA rests on the passages in Meditation Six where Descartes talks about true errors of nature, this defense is weak.

I conclude that, even if TA did offer an account of representational content, it is not obvious that it would provide a solution to the puzzle of misrepresentation. I will close this chapter by arguing that TA lacks strong textual support.

[38] This objection was made by Don Garrett at a meeting of New York/New Jersey Workshop in Early Modern Philosophy. Garrett's reading is reinforced by Descartes' conclusions, in Meditation Six, that "notwithstanding the immense goodness of God, the nature of man as a combination of mind and body is such that it is bound to mislead him from time to time. For there may be some occurrence, not in the foot but in one of the other areas through which the nerves travel in their route from the foot to the brain, or even in the brain itself; and if this cause produces the same motion which is generally produced by the injury in the foot, the pain will be felt as if it were in the foot. *This deception of the senses is natural*, because a given motion in the brain must always produce the same motion in the mind; and the origin of the motion in question is much more often going to be something which is hurting the foot, rather than something existing elsewhere" (CSM II 61; AT VII 88, emphasis added). Notice that here the occasional deceptiveness of the senses is said to be *natural* not because it is a deviation from the proper purpose of the senses, but because, despite God's institution of a law-like correspondence between mental states and bodily states, the nature of man as a combination of mind and body is bound to disrupt (at times) this law-like correspondence.

4.4 AN ALTERNATIVE READING OF THE TELEOLOGICAL JARGON OF MEDITATION SIX

Meditation Six, according to Simmons, provides the best support for TA. In my view, however, all Descartes claims in Meditation Six is that the *information* carried by sensations can be *used* by the mind–body union to avoid what's harmful and seek out what's beneficial. Descartes opens the discussion of sensation by claiming that "there is no doubt that everything that I am taught by nature [read: the mind–body union] contains *some* truth (*et sane non dubium est quin ea omnia quae doceor a nature aliquid hebeant veritatis*)" (CSM II 56, my emphasis; AT VII 80). Notice that the expression *aliquid veritatis* (some truth) suggests that the senses provide a *partially correct representation* of things. And their representation is *partially* correct because sensations do represent existing things (as we assume uncritically) although they misrepresent them (since sensations do not resemble the properties they represent).[39] Further down, Descartes is quite explicit about what is the *partial* truth the senses convey:

> [. . .] although I feel heat when I go near a fire and feel pain when I go too near, there is no convincing argument for supposing there is something in the fire which resembles the heat [. . .]. There is simply reason to suppose that there is *something* in the fire, *whatever it may eventually turn out to be, which produces in us* the feelings of heat and pain. (CSM II 57; AT VII 83, emphasis added)

So, according to Descartes, *first* sensations teach us that there are bodies existing in our vicinity. From the fact that we perceive a variety of colors, smells, tastes, shapes and so on, we can infer that "the bodies which are the source of the various sensory perceptions possess differences corresponding to them, though perhaps not resembling them" (CSM II 56; AT VII 81). And *then* he adds: "Also (*Atque*) the fact that some of the perceptions are agreeable to me while others are disagreeable makes it quite certain that my body [. . .] can be affected by various beneficial or harmful

[39] Notice, incidentally, that if Simmons were right, Descartes shouldn't have written that sensations contain *some* truth; he should have said that sensations (as Simmons suggests) are "materially true" since they fulfill the purpose for which they were bestowed on us (*viz.*, they secure the survival of the mind–body union).

bodies which surround it" (Ibid.). The "atque" suggests that the *information about*, or representation of, bodies *carried by* sensations can *moreover* ("atque") be *used* to seek out or avoid the objects that are, respectively, beneficial or harmful to the man. Needless to say, these objects couldn't be pursued or avoided unless they were *already* represented.

There is, however, the passage where Descartes writes that "the *proper purpose* of sensory perceptions [. . .] is simply to inform the mind of what is beneficial or harmful for the composite. But [we] *misuse* them by treating them as reliable touchstones for immediate judgments about the essential natures of the bodies located outside us" (CSM II 57–58, emphasis added; AT VII 83). This passage provides the strongest support for Simmons' interpretation since it suggests that the senses are designed to secure the survival of the mind–body union and, hence, that they represent what they do in virtue of their biological function. But this is an exaggerated reading of the text.

Claiming that the proper purpose of the senses is to inform the mind of what's beneficial or harmful to the mind–body union isn't necessarily equivalent to claiming that sensations represent what they do in virtue of their biological function. Fulfillment of this purpose is compatible with an alternative account of what makes sensations represent what they do. When Descartes writes that "the proper purpose of the senses is to inform the mind of what is beneficial or harmful to the composite" he may be just repeating what he had already said, namely, that the senses represent existing bodies around us and *because of this* their *proper* purpose (*as opposed to* the purpose of discovering the true nature of reality) is to promote the man's well-being. Accordingly, we would be misusing sensations by treating them as reliable indicators of the true essence of bodies.

One may still raise the following concern regarding this reading of Meditation Six. Certainly, the objection goes, the composite makes use of sensations quite automatically or unconsciously. This fact suggests that the biological function is built into sensations and so some kind of natural teleology is reintroduced.[40] To answer this objection we need to distinguish two claims. The first claim is that *sensations serve the biological function of preserving the health of the composite.* The second claim is that *sensations represent what they do in virtue of the biological function of*

[40] This objection was raised in different contexts by Lilli Alanen and Sean Greenberg.

preserving the health of the composite. It is undeniable that Descartes endorsed the first claim. But the finality of sensation may simply be parasitic on the fact that sensations represent what they do quite independently of their purpose. In fact, it may be the case that sensations give rise quite automatically to behavior that promotes the survival of the mind–body union *because* they are by and large veridical.[41] Notice that Descartes in Meditation Six does seem to suggest this when he writes that "I am taught by nature that various objects exist in the vicinity of my body *and* that some of these are to be sought out and others to be avoided" (CSM II 56; AT VII 81, emphasis added); and that "[m]y nature [. . .] does indeed teach me to avoid what *induces* a feeling of pain and seek out what induces feelings of pleasure" (CSM II 57; AT VII 82, emphasis added). Both passages suggest that, according to Descartes, sensations represent objects *first* in a non-evaluative way; and *then* such representations *induce* feelings of pain, desire, repulsion, fear. It is in virtue of what they represent that they are naturally used to seek out what's beneficial and avoid what's harmful. And, so, it is possible to acknowledge that, according to Descartes, the composite makes use of sensations automatically without attributing to him the view that sensations represent what they do in virtue of their biological role.

CONCLUSIONS

For all the above reasons, I conclude that TA is not Descartes' considered position. Besides the fact that the texts do not clearly support it, the theoretical costs of TA are too high to be negotiated for its benefits. Moreover, it is not even clear that TA has these benefits. TA is supposed to be an improvement on CA. However, TA inherits some of the same problems that CA was already diagnosed to have (for example, the problem of presupposing rather than providing an account of representational content); it fails to provide a straightforward solution to these problems (for example, the problem of misrepresentation); and it introduces more theoretical difficulties for Descartes than it solves.

[41] The fact that an object can be quite naturally used for a certain purpose does not necessarily imply that it was made for that purpose.

5

A Descriptivist-Causal Account and the Solution of the Puzzle of Sensory Representation

Cartesian sensations are representational and their representational content is neither the result of a judgment nor the result of purely external relations with the environment. Chapter 3 concluded that CA's failures indicate that representationality must be an internal property of sensations and that there are theoretical and textual grounds for this reading. In this chapter, I offer a detailed defense of this conclusion.

I will defend a *qualified* internalist account of the representationality of Cartesian sensations. Although I maintain that sensations represent what they do in virtue of some internal feature (along the lines of DA), I also argue that a causal relation to bodily states plays a role in the formation of sensory ideas of color and the like. I will call my account "descriptivist-causal" to differentiate it from purely internalist accounts and I will argue that this account has the advantage, over the latter, of not only acknowledging all those texts where Descartes explicitly claims that ideas of sense are caused by bodies in us, but also of explaining what distinguishes sensory representation from purely intellectual representation. Purely internalist accounts overlook these texts and, so, fail to provide a satisfactory account of *sensory* representation. Purely causal accounts overplay (and misinterpret) these texts and end up with an altogether mistaken account of the *representationality* of Cartesian sensations. My descriptivist-causal account, instead, provides a reading of these texts that allows us to incorporate the role of the mind's causal interaction with body within an overall internalist account of the representationality of sensation while accounting for the distinguishing feature of sensory representation (*viz.*, the fact that sensations represent their objects as other than they are).

I will start with a discussion of currently available purely internalist accounts of Cartesian sensations (5.1); then I will proceed to defend my descriptivist-causal account (5.2–5.6) and explain how it solves the puzzle of sensory misrepresentation (5.7).

5.1 PURELY INTERNALIST ACCOUNTS

Although an internalist reading of the representationality of Cartesian sensations is not popular, it has some supporters. In this section, I will present Martha Bolton's and Andrew Pessin's internalist accounts and discuss what I take to be their limitations and difficulties.[1]

Andrew Pessin's argument for an internalist reading of the representationality of Cartesian sensations runs as follows. According to Descartes, ideas have a two-fold nature. They are essentially related to us (insofar as they are conscious states) but they are also essentially representing an object to the mind (in virtue of their objective reality). So the (non-reflective) awareness of an idea is the direct awareness of the object of the idea.[2] Let the object of thought be an external object. Accordingly, as Descartes claims in his exchange with Caterus, the intellectual idea of the sun "is the sun itself existing in the intellect" (CSM II 75; AT VII 103).[3] Once Pessin has established this point for intellectual ideas, he goes on to make the same argument for sensory ideas:

> Just as Fred's thought of the sun just *is* the sun, so too sensation-y [read: Fred's state of sensing yellow] *is* motion-m [read: a particular type of primary qualities causing the sensation], sensed. Just as Fred's direct (i.e., non reflective) awareness of his thinking of the sun just *is* his (cognitively) direct awareness of the sun, so, too, Fred's direct (i.e., non reflective) awareness of his sensing of yellow just is his (cognitively) direct awareness of motion-m. In sensing the yellow, Fred is in fact sensing motion-m (despite his not realizing it).[4]

[1] See Bolton (1986) and (2002); and Pessin (2009).

[2] For Descartes' distinction between awareness and reflective awareness see CSM I 122; AT VI 23; CSMK 335; AT V 149; CSM II 128; AT VII 182–183.

[3] Pessin explains that Descartes must be discussing the intellectual idea of the sun, that is, "the sun in so far as we are [...] thinking about it on the basis of astronomical reasoning. [...] Such an idea would involve clear and distinct ideas of extension and its modes" (Pessin (2009), p. 3, fn. 10; see also pp. 5–9).

[4] Ibid., pp. 9–10, original emphasis.

The driving *assumption* is that sensations are modeled after the intellectual ideas of external things – where intellectual ideas are the paradigm representational states. And since intellectual ideas represent their objects intrinsically or in virtue of internal features (as opposed to in virtue of external relations) so must sensations. Here's why:

> Suppose [. . .] that sensation-y represented motion-m by virtue of some external relation between y and m. If so, then Fred's awareness of his state of sensing would be hard to identify with his awareness of m, since nothing about that state itself (or awareness thereof) would contain or indicate m. Indeed, if nothing intrinsic to his sensing yellow indicates m, Fred would not be said to be sensing m at all. [So] [. . .] the representational property [of sensation] [must] be an intrinsic or internal one: something about sensation-y *intrinsically* makes it a representation of motion-m. [In the case of intellectual ideas there is] an internal relation between the idea and its *representandum*. We ought not to demand anything different from sensory ideas.[5]

So, according to Pessin, Fred would *not be said to be sensing m* at all unless *something intrinsic to his sensing yellow indicates m.* Given that Pessin acknowledges the epistemic role of ideas in Descartes' philosophy and writes explicitly that "Fred's direct (i.e., non reflective) awareness of his sensing of yellow just is his (cognitively) direct awareness of motion-m," I take it that Pessin means that Fred could not be said to sense m at all unless something intrinsic to his sensing yellow *cognitively* indicates m.

A complication arises due to an acknowledged disanalogy between sensory and intellectual ideas. Pessin admits that in the case of sensations – unlike in the case of intellectual ideas – we must "distinguish between sensations being representational and our being able to determine that (and what) they represent."[6] This is a necessary concession, Pessin admits, because sensations are obscure and confused ideas and, so, represent their correct objects although we may not have epistemic access to them (i.e., the objects).

So, we have a problem. Given that, according to Pessin, one could not be said to sense an external object unless something intrinsic to the sensation cognitively indicated this object, either we conclude that sensations are not representational altogether and, so, that in sensing yellow

[5] Ibid., p. 13, original emphasis.
[6] Ibid., p. 12.

Fred is not sensing m at all; or we conclude, along the lines of externalist accounts, that in the case of sensations the epistemic dimension of representation is lost. Sensations represent what they do in virtue of causal relations of which the subject may be totally ignorant. But Pessin does not want to endorse either conclusion. Instead, he wants to say that sensations are representational *and* that they are internally representational. Wishing to avoid either one of the above conclusions, but unable to explain why sensations still (*cognitively*) *intrinsically* represent an object to the mind, he is cornered in drawing the unsatisfactory conclusion that sensory representation "is a primitive for Descartes."[7]

Pessin's conclusion is deeply unsatisfying. It taints his internalist account since, in fact, *no* internalist account of sensory representation is provided. It is a contradiction to claim that there must be "something about sensation-y [that] *intrinsically* makes it a representation of motion-m"[8] and, at the same time, to claim that sensory representation is a primitive since "there may be nothing about a sensation to which we could point and say 'that is the feature by virtue of which it represents.'"[9] One may argue that since Pessin insists that the sensation *internally* represents its objects even if we are unable to determine what it is, an *explanation* of how the sensation internally represents its object is in order. Saying that it is a primitive does not help. Besides, notice that a supporter of a causal theory could object that a sensation represents its right objects even if we are unable to tell what it is simply *because it is caused by it* in the right way. Since Pessin denies that Descartes held a causal theory, an internalist *explanation* of how sensations represent their right objects is necessary on pain of simply begging the question with supporters of a causal reading. The burden of proof is on the internalist and Pessin fails to provide any satisfactory answer.

Sometimes Pessin seems to suggest that no explanation of how sensations intrinsically represent their objects is necessary because even in the case of intellectual ideas no such explanation is needed. Descartes, that is, would have no account whatsoever of mental

[7] Pessin (2009), p. 14 and p. 24.
[8] Ibid., p. 13.
[9] Ibid., p. 14.

representation.[10] But Descartes *does* have an account of mental representation. Ideas, according to Descartes, are mental states that are "as it were the images of things" (CSM II 25; AT VII 37) and, as Normore has pointed out, there was a long scholastic tradition of explaining the representationality of ideas or their objective being through the analogy with images.[11] Since not all ideas are the product of the imagination for Descartes, the analogy ought not to be taken literally. Descartes means to say that ideas represent by providing an identifying description of the object of thought and that the referent of the idea is what satisfies such description (see Chapter 1 above). So, Pessin is wrong even when it comes to intellectual ideas. Descartes does have an account of mental representation. And in the case of sensory ideas, the need for explaining why the sensation of yellow represents a certain configuration of matter becomes even more pressing. Why? Because there is an epistemic difference between sensory and intellectual ideas. The latter contain a clear and distinct and, hence, identifying description of the object of thought. The former do not. Pessin repeats this over and over again:

> Strictly speaking, the object of sensation-y, [on my account], just is motion-m; y just *is* m, sensed. The problem is that y on its own fails to allow Fred to determine the true nature of y's object. Suppose, then, that the right sort of correspondence were partly governed by epistemic needs. [. . .] [I]f so, an idea would *resemble* its object if and only if the true nature of its object were epistemically accessible to the agent on the basis of the idea alone. [So, on my account] sensation y fails to resemble motion-m in so far as we cannot determine visually that its object is m. But that is perfectly consistent with m's actually being y's object.[12]

But saying that (given the lack of resemblance between the qualitative aspect of experience and the object of the idea) we cannot determine *visually* the object of the idea is not only consistent with motion-m being the object of sensation y (as Pessin correctly notices) but it is also consistent with an internalist *explanation* of why this is so. That's what Pessin misses. As we shall see below (5.6), my own account provides the missing explanation of why sensations represent their correct objects *internally* even if the qualitative character of experience makes it

[10] Ibid., p. 26.
[11] See Normore (1986).
[12] Pessin (2009), p. 28, original emphasis. See also pp. 29–30.

difficult for us to determine what these objects are. By providing this missing explanation, my account, unlike Pessin's, is a genuine internalist account.

The seeds of a much more promising internalist account can be found (somewhat implicitly) in Bolton (1986) and (more explicitly) in Bolton (2002).[13] Martha Bolton argues that an intelligible content, hidden in sensory ideas, is responsible for the representationality of sensations. Since the intelligible content is such that it exhibits the true object of the idea (in the case of the idea of red, for example, a particular type of configuration of particles having primary qualities); and this object (due to the doctrine of the transparency of thought) cannot be totally "veiled from recognition;" the idea of red exhibits an unknown quality of body in virtue of this semi-hidden intelligible content. As Bolton puts it, "a false idea (or any confused, obscure idea) represents by means that are not evident from the idea itself."[14] And this explanation of the initial representationality of sensory ideas finds support in the Cartesian doctrine (sketched in the *Regulae ad Directionem Ingenii* and in the *Principles*) that every thought is composed of primitive simple notions that determine its intentional content.[15]

In Bolton's view, then, the presence of a hidden intellectual/intelligible content *both* explains why ideas of sense initially seem to represent qualities of bodies *and* determines what these ideas actually represent (that is, a particular configuration of particles of matter having primary

[13] In neither Bolton (1986) nor Bolton (2002) is Martha Bolton's primary target an explicit defense of an internalist reading of Cartesian sensations and, so, her views are not as explicitly presented as I make them out to be. However, I take it that the following presentation of Bolton's view is a fair rendition of what she would say if she were asked to express a view on this issue. My understanding of Bolton's view benefited from numerous conversations with her.

[14] See Bolton (1986), p. 395.

[15] This is made explicit in Bolton (2002). In the original article (that was written in English and is unpublished), Bolton writes: "[...] some of Descartes' statements hint that sensory ideas have intentional content that may be initially hidden [...]. [His view is that sensory ideas have] minimal intelligible content [...]. I want to suggest that there are resources for explicating the notion of hidden intentional [or intelligible] content in Descartes' theory that all thoughts are constituted of simple notions and that we arrive at true judgments by clarifying the simple notions judgments contain. This [...] speculative psychological doctrine of Descartes [...] underwrites a picture on which thoughts or ideas, whether confused or not, are composed of (contain) basic simple notions that determine their intentional content."

qualities). Accordingly, the intentional content of sensory ideas is *internally* determined because it is the mind that conceptualizes the object of, for example, the idea of red as a certain type of configuration of matter that corresponds to (and is the cause of) the idea.

I agree with Bolton's suggestion that a latent intellectual/intelligible content explains the intentionality of sensations and I develop it further below (5.2). However, unlike Bolton, I maintain that a purely internalist account fails to provide an accurate account of *sensory* representation and, hence, fails to explain the phenomenon of sensory misrepresentation.[16] The nature of my disagreement with Bolton can be summarized as follows. It is only *after* a (reflective) process of clarification and analysis of the confused sensory content (in light of the clear and distinct idea of matter) that ideas of sense can be said to represent a certain type of configuration of matter.[17] This type of configuration of matter is what satisfies the *clarified* content of the idea. But this is *not* what sensory ideas represent. They represent obscurely, that is, they represent configurations of matter as resembling the sensation. And a purely internalist account based on the notion of a latent intelligible content alone *cannot* explain this phenomenon. Besides, if what determines the content of sensory ideas is only the intelligible content coming from the simple notions, how can we account for the fact that a sensory idea represents one object or one type of configuration of matter rather than another? After all, the intelligible understanding of the object of thought can only give us an understanding of the essential properties of matter and hence it would fail to distinguish one material object from another. I will return to a discussion of these points in sections 5.5 and 5.6 below.

For different reasons, then, currently available internalist accounts are not fully satisfactory explanations of Descartes' views on sensory representation. In the following sections (5.2–5.5), I will defend a *qualified* internalist account, *viz.*, a descriptivist-causal account. This account preserves the internalist intuition that the object of sensation is determined by something intrinsic to the sensation itself but develops this intuition into a more elaborate account that, among other things, explains what distinguishes *sensory* from intellectual representation.

[16] I used to disagree with Bolton's account for different reasons. See De Rosa (2004).
[17] On this, see De Rosa (2004).

I will begin, in 5.2 below, by defending in more detail my earlier claim (see Chapter 3) that representationality must be an *internal* property of sensation.

5.2 THE INTERNALIST ELEMENT IN SENSORY REPRESENTATION

At the end of Chapter 3, I drew the interim conclusion that the representationality of sensory ideas must come from the mind itself. The problems raised for causal accounts indicated that, according to Descartes, bodies can be regarded as causes of sensory ideas only insofar as they are *already* represented *as* bodies. But it remains to be explained why the object of the sensory idea is already conceived *as* a body. My suggestion at the end of Chapter 3 was that the representationality comes from the innate ideas of body and extension which are present in sensory representation despite the fact that we may not be aware of them. In this section, I defend this suggestion in more detail.

I argued elsewhere that, according to Descartes, the mind contains innate ideas neither in the sense that the mind is aware of them since birth nor in the sense that the mind is disposed to acquire them in life. Rather, innate ideas are ideas that the mind contains without being (fully) aware of them.[18] Although this reading of innate ideas may be at odds with Descartes' doctrine of the transparency of thought, a number of scholars have acknowledged that Descartes is nonetheless committed to it.[19] Attempts have been made to resolve the inconsistency by appealing to Descartes' distinction between implicit and explicit knowledge and unreflective and reflective cognition.[20] The question of whether Descartes has

[18] Notice that the latter claim is *not* equivalent to the claim that the mind possesses some general learning mechanism that disposes it to acquire ideas because it implies that the mind is *already predisposed* to learn certain types of ideas (rather than others) as a result of encounters with the environment. We learn (from the environment) what was, so to speak, already in us – even if we were not fully aware of it. On this see De Rosa (2004a).

[19] On this see Wilson (1978), pp. 150–165.

[20] For example, one may argue that x can have either implicit or non-reflective knowledge, but still no actual knowledge of an idea. And there are certainly passages where Descartes seems to suggest this reading of innateness. But there are also other passages where innate ideas are said not to be known until we have explicit awareness of

the theoretical resources for resolving this *prima facie* inconsistency is an interesting exegetical question. But I do not need to take a stand on it in this context. All that matters here is that Descartes believed that the mind contains innate ideas of which the mind is not immediately aware and that these ideas constitute the inner structure of our thoughts insofar as they "shape" our particular thoughts. As Leibniz would put it, these ideas "are necessary for thought as muscles and tendons are for walking."[21] As the structure of muscles and tendons is what allows us to walk the way we do (although we are not aware of them), so innate ideas and principles allow us to think the way we do. And insofar as these ideas and principles constitute the structure of our thoughts, the mind must be (at least) *minimally* aware of them. It is this aspect of Descartes' theory of innate ideas that I want to emphasize for our purposes.

In a few places, for example, Descartes suggests that the innate ideas of thought and existence and the general principle "whatever thinks exists" are present in the particular thought "I think therefore I am" although we are not fully aware of their presence.[22] In Meditation Three, Descartes claims that the proposition "I think therefore I am" is the first item of knowledge.[23] But in Principles I.10, he also claims that the primitiveness of the proposition "I think therefore I exist" does not rule out "that one must *first know* what thought, existence and certainty are, and that it is impossible that that which thinks should not exist, and so forth" (CSM I 196; AT VIIIA 8, emphasis added). In reply to Burman's queries, Descartes explains:

Before this inference, "I am thinking, therefore I exist," the major "whatever thinks exists" can be known; for it is in reality prior to my inference, and my

them. On this debate, see, for example, McRae (1972) and Wilson (1978), pp. 150–165. For Descartes' distinctions between implicit and explicit knowledge and unreflective and reflective cognition, see for example, CSMK 333; AT V 147; and CSM II 285; AT VII 422.

[21] Leibniz (1996), pp. 83–84.

[22] For evidence that Descartes regards the ideas of thought and existence as innate see, for example, CSM II 285; AT VII 422; CSM II 26; AT VII 38. For evidence that Descartes regards the general principle "Whatever thinks exists" as innate see Principles I.49 (where Descartes lists this principle among the eternal truths) and for the innateness of all eternal truths see, for example, CSMK 23; AT I 145.

[23] See CSM II 24; AT VII 35. See also CSM II 100; AT VII 140 and *Letter to Clerselier*, June or July 1646 (CSMK 290; AT IV 445).

inference depends on it. That is why the author says in the Principles that the major premises comes first, namely because *implicitly* it is always presupposed and prior. But it does not follow that I am always *expressly and explicitly aware* of its priority, or that I know it before by inference. This is because I am attending only to what I experience within myself – for example, "I am thinking, therefore I exist". I do not pay attention in the same way to the general notion "whatever thinks exists". [...] *we do not separate out* these general propositions from the particular instances; rather, *it is in the particular instances that we think of them.* (CSMK 333; AT V 147, emphasis added. See also CSM II 285; AT VII 422)

Descartes is saying that in experiencing the particular thought "I think therefore I am" one may fail to pay attention to the general principle "Whatever thinks exists" and the innate ideas of thought and existence, although the principle and ideas are *not separate* from the particular thought. We think of the general principles and innate ideas *in their particular instances* although the former are always (psychologically) prior to, and presupposed by, the latter.

More generally, consider that Descartes' simple notions correspond to innate ideas. The simple notions that Descartes lists in a letter to Princess Elizabeth (CSMK 226; AT III 691) and in the *Principles* (CSM I 208–209; AT VIIIA 22–23)[24] are said to be innate in other places. The ideas of body and mind are called "innate," for example, in Meditation Two (CSM II 21; AT VII 31), in the *Regulae* (CSM I 44; AT X 419), and in a letter to Mersenne (CSMK 183; AT III 383); the "common" simple notions of existence, being, duration are called "innate" in the Sixth Set of Replies (CSM II 285; AT VII 422), Meditation Three (CSM II 26; AT VII 38) and, in Meditation Five, the duration we assign to motions is said to be "in harmony with my nature" (CSM II 44; AT VII 64). According to Descartes, the simple notions are "the basic components of our thought" (CSM I 208; AT VIIIA 22), "the patterns on the basis of which we form all our conceptions" (CSMK 218; AT III 665).[25] As he claims in Meditation One, in the passages where he discusses the painter analogy, we must admit that "certain [...] even simpler and more universal things [that is, 'corporeal nature in nature, and its extension; the shape of extended things; the

[24] Notice that this list corresponds roughly to the list of simple natures of the *Regulae ad Directionem Ingenii* (CSM I 44–45; AT X 419).

[25] See also CSM I 46; AT X 422.

quantity, or size and number of these things'] are real. These are, as it were, the real colours from which we form all the images of things, whether true or false, that occur in our thought" (CSM II 14; AT VII 20). This confirms that innate ideas, according to Descartes, are present (although latently) in all our particular thoughts and determine their contents by giving them an intentional object. Descartes' exchange with Gassendi on the innate idea of triangle illustrates perfectly the sense in which innate ideas structure, for example, the content of our sensory perceptions. Descartes writes:

> [. . .] since the idea of a true triangle was already in us, and could be conceived by our minds more easily than the composite figure we did not apprehend the figure we saw, but rather the true triangle. It is just the same as when we look at a piece of paper on which some lines have been drawn in ink to represent a man's face: the idea that this produces in us is not so much the idea of these lines as the idea of a man. Yet this would certainly not happen unless the human face were already known to us from some other source, and we were more accustomed to think of the face than the lines drawn in ink [. . .]. Thus we could not recognize the geometrical triangle from the diagram on the paper unless our mind already possessed the idea of it from some other source. (CSM II 262; AT VII 382)

Descartes claims that the presence of the idea of triangle in the mind is what allows us to *see* and *recognize* particular triangles, that is, it is what allows us to have the sensory perception *of* a particular triangle.[26]

Descartes' views on the role of the innate ideas of body and its categorial features (such as extension, size, shape etc.) in our sensory perception of particular bodies are clear in the famous discussion of the piece of wax in Meditation Two. Descartes begins the discussion by noticing that although all the features of the piece of wax that are known by the senses change when the wax is put by the fire, we still perceive the *same* wax. Then he goes on to ask: "So what was in the wax that I understood with such distinctness" (CSM II 20; AT VII 30)? The

[26] Also, in the *Optics*, Descartes argues that the perception of the distance (and, hence, size and shape) of bodies requires the use of some kind of "natural geometry (*geometrie naturelle*)" (CSM I 170; AT VI 137). Although he also says that this calculation "is done by a mental act which [is] only a very simple act of the imagination" (CSM I 170; AT VI 138) he does not deny that the calculation involves a reasoning that presumably resorts to some innate geometrical principles and ideas. This is compatible with Descartes' view that geometrical knowledge is aided by the imagination although it is not fully explained by it.

answer is that we distinctly perceive the wax *as a body having extension and capable of endless changes in figure and shape* and that such distinct perception comes from the intellect alone ("I must therefore admit that the nature of this piece of wax is [. . .] perceived by the mind alone" CSM II 21; AT VII 31). But, immediately afterwards, Descartes clarifies that "this wax which is perceived by the mind alone" (Ibid.) "is the same wax which I see, which I touch [. . .] in short the same wax which I thought it to be from the start" (Ibid.). I take Descartes to be saying here that the distinct (and intellectual) perception of the wax *as a body having certain categorial features* is latently contained (and actively employed) in the confused sensory perception of the piece of wax. This is confirmed by Descartes' explanation that our perception of the piece of wax is a matter of mental scrutiny that "can be imperfect and confused, as it was before, or clear and distinct as it is now, just as I attend more or less attentively on the elements of which it is composed (*prout minus vel magis ad illa ex quibus constat attendo*)" (CSM II 21; AT VII 3).[27] It is in virtue of this intellectual but latent perception that we *see* the piece of wax as always the same (as an enduring body under different appearances) and, *hence*, we are inclined to *judge* that the same piece of wax is in front of us.

My view is that the case of ideas of red and the like is similar to the case of the idea of the piece of wax. As we saw in Chapter 2, there is neither textual evidence nor sound argument that supports the view that our perceptions of secondary qualities are either non-representational or represent *qualia*. On the contrary, we saw that in several places Descartes includes perceptions of secondary qualities among ideas of corporeal things. Perceptions of red and the like represent bodies (albeit confusedly). But the pressing question was: in virtue of what do they represent them given that the phenomenal red (say) does not resemble any corporeal property? In Chapters 3 and 4, I argued that neither a causal nor a teleofunctional theory can explain this feature of sensory ideas. I suggested that the representationality exhibited by sensory ideas must come from something internal to the sensory idea itself. Now I have the theoretical resources to substantiate this suggestion. The

[27] Notice that my translation here differs from Cottingham's translation. The latter, in my view, fails to bring out the meaning of "being composed of" carried by the Latin verb "*consto*."

innate ideas of body and its categorial features are as latently present in our perception of secondary qualities as they are in our perception of the piece of wax. It is the presence of this latent intellectual content that makes our perception of secondary qualities ideas *of* bodies. As our perception of the wax *as* something extended behind the mutable sensory appearances is to be explained in virtue of the hidden intellectual perception of the wax, so our experience of red *as* a property of body is also to be explained in virtue of some latent intellectual content.[28] Besides, since the innate ideas of body and its categorial features are the ideas that structure our knowledge of the physical world and our knowledge of the physical world does originate in (although it is not exhausted by) sensory perception, it is inevitable that the mind employs these innate ideas in the sensory apprehension of the external world. Consequently, the mind is bound to experience sensory appearances *as properties of the physical world.*

Let me conclude this section with further textual evidence in support of my reading of the intentionality of sensory ideas. In several places Descartes writes that it is the same mind which understands, imagines, remembers and has sensory perceptions. In Meditation Six, he writes:

> [...] I find in myself faculties for certain special modes of thinking, namely imagination and sensory perception. Now I can clearly and distinctly perceive myself as a whole without these faculties; but I cannot, conversely, understand these faculties without *me*, that is, without *an intellectual substance* to inhere in. This is because there is *an intellectual act* included in their essential definition. (CSM II 54; AT VII 78, emphasis added)

Descartes claims here that intellection is the essential feature of the thinking thing or mind.[29] This claim does not deny that imagination and sensory perceptions are modes of the thinking substance. It does imply, however, that the intellect enters, so to speak, *any* mode of thought. Any mode of the thinking substance, including imagination and sensory perception, is (in some sense) an intellectual act ("[...]

[28] Notice that Descartes' claim, in *Comments on a Certain Broadsheet*, that the ideas of pain and the like are innate because there is no similarity between the cause and the content of the ideas (CSM I 304; AT VIIIB 359) is at least compatible with my claim that the content of sensory ideas "contains" some implicit intellectual content.

[29] This was already the interim conclusion of Meditation Two: "I am then [...] a mind, or intelligence, or intellect, or reason [...]" (CSM II 18; AT VII 27).

there is an intellectual act included in [the] essential definition [of imagination and sensory perception]"). Descartes repeats this view in the *Principles*, where he writes that "sensory perception, imagination and pure understanding are simply various modes of perception" (CSM I 204; AT VIIIA 17) and that perception is an "operation of the intellect" (Ibid.) According to Descartes, every substance has one principal attribute and every mode of that substance presupposes such attribute.[30] So, Descartes is claiming that *thought* in the sense of *intellection* is the essential property, or principal attribute, of the mind. Hence, every mode of the mind presupposes intellection.[31] All mental acts are operations of the intellect.

But what does Descartes mean by "intellect" here? Clearly it cannot be the intellect as the faculty of pure understanding (or understanding clearly and distinctly) since "understanding" is only one of the listed operations of the intellect. So what is this faculty of the intellect more broadly construed? Now consider that the mark of the mental, besides consciousness, is the property of representationality for Descartes.[32] Thoughts, besides being conscious states, have intentional objects. It follows that the intellect, broadly construed as a faculty of representation, is responsible for the intentionality exhibited by all mental states. *But, as we saw in our above discussion, it is the innate ideas or simple notions contained in the intellect that determine the intentional content of our thoughts.* So it is the intellect as a faculty endowed with specific innate ideas (as opposed to some bare faculty) that unifies the mental

[30] Principles I.53, CSM I 210; AT VIII A 25.

[31] Here's a similar passage from the *Regulae*: "[The cognitive power] is one and the same power: when applying itself along with the imagination to the "common" sense, it is said to see, touch etc.; when addressing itself to the imagination alone, in so far as the latter is invested with various figures, it is said to remember; when applying itself to the imagination in order to form new figures, it is said to imagine or conceive; and lastly when it acts on its own, it is said to understand. [...] According to its different functions, then, the same power is called either pure intellect, or imagination, or memory, or sensory perception" (CSM I 42; AT X 415–416). Now if the cognitive power is the same in understanding, imagining and sensing and an intellectual act is contained in the essential definition of not only understanding but also of imagination and sensory perception then the cognitive power which is the same in every operation of the mind is the intellect.

[32] See Descartes' Second Set of Replies CSM II 113–114 (definitions I–III); AT VII 160–161; Meditation Three, CSM II 25–26; AT VII 37; and Descartes' claim in Meditation Three that "there can be no ideas that are not as it were of things" (CSM I 30; AT VII 44). On this see Hatfield (2003), pp. 258–259.

and constitutes the essential feature of the thinking mind. Notice that claiming that the intellect as a faculty endowed with specific innate ideas constitutes the essential feature of the thinking mind implies neither a denial of Descartes' claim that all mental states are essentially conscious states nor "an intellectualization" of sensory representation.[33] It only implies that the same innate ideas or notions are included in every mental event, although in different ways. When the mind turns inwards and examines its own ideas it is said to understand or to "intellect" in a pure way, but when it turns toward the body, it is said to imagine and have sensations. The employment of innate ideas in our sensory perception does not *intellectualize* it since the senses have their own way of representing bodies to us and may resort to all sorts of different empirical cues (besides conceptual ones) to accomplish this. My view only implies that these ideas or simple notions structure the phenomenological appearance of the external world by allowing us to *conceptualize* the objects of our sensory experience.

Having established that sensory experience is representational insofar as it essentially includes an intellectual act, I want now to shift attention to another important Cartesian claim, namely, Descartes' view that sensations are modes of the mind–body union and hence, in some sense are products of the mind's causal interaction with bodies. In particular, I want to focus on this question: in what sense, if any, does the causal interaction with bodies, or properties thereof, affect Descartes' theory of sensory representation? I will address this question in the following two sections.

5.3 THE ROLE OF THE CAUSAL CONNECTION IN SENSORY REPRESENTATION: THE ALLEGED EVIDENCE FROM MEDITATION SIX

The causal reading of the representationality of Cartesian sensations is often defended on a textual basis.[34] Since the argument for the existence of

[33] For this complaint see Simmons (2003). It is not clear what Simmons means by this but I take it that it implies that the senses would be deprived of their *own way* of representing the world. I will return to this issue in Chapter 6 below.

[34] See especially Schmaltz (1992) and (2006); Hoffman (1996); and, to a certain extent, De Rosa (2004). I left the discussion of this textual evidence to this chapter

material things in Meditation Six is alleged to provide the best support for a causal reading, I will begin with a discussion of this argument.

In Meditation Six, Descartes writes that the faculty of sensory perception is a passive faculty "for receiving (*recipiendi*) and recognizing (*cognoscendi*) the ideas of sensible objects"[35] (CSM II 55; AT VII 79). In order to explain this passive reception, we need to search for "an active faculty, either in me or in something else, which produced or brought about these ideas" (Ibid.). Descartes argues that this active faculty cannot be either the mind as a purely intellectual faculty (since the *reception* of sensory ideas "clearly presupposes no intellectual act on my part" (Ibid.)) or the will (since "the ideas in questions are produced without my cooperation and often against my will' (Ibid.)).[36] God would be a deceiver if he caused these ideas in us since we *have a propensity to believe* that they come from external bodies. The only possible conclusion is that this active faculty consists of material bodies. This proves that body, or corporeal nature, exists as the cause of our ideas.

This argument, according to supporters of a causal reading, is an implicit defense of a causal account of sensations as follows. Since what is at stake, in the above argument, is the explanation of why ideas of sense exhibit objective reality (*viz.*, represent bodies), the conclusion that bodies are the causes of our ideas of sense *would imply* that bodies are the causes of the objective reality of sensory ideas. Sensory ideas represent bodies because they are caused by bodies and the explicit use

(rather than discussing it in Chapter 3) because I find it more appropriate to examine it in the context of the question I am addressing now, that is: Given the arguments of Chapter 3, but in light of the fact that Descartes regards sensations as products of the mind's causal interaction with bodies, in what sense, *if any*, does the causal interaction with bodies affect Descartes' theory of sensory representation?

[35] Curiously enough the ability to "recognize" ideas of sensible objects does not seem to imply passivity. I won't focus on this detail here but it is interesting to notice that, according to Descartes, the overall passive character of sensory perception may not rule out an active role of the mind.

[36] Notice that the claim that the active faculty cannot be the mind as an intellectual faculty because the reception of sensory ideas "presupposes no intellectual act on my part" does not contradict the claim made earlier on in Meditation Six that there is an intellectual act included in the essential definition of sensory perception (CSM II 54; AT VII 78). What Descartes is interested in emphasizing here is that the faculty of sensory perception is not the function of the pure (or disembodied) mind. One of the conclusions that Meditation Six establishes is that sensations are the product of the union of the mind with the body.

of the causal principle in the proof would warrant this reasoning. Schmaltz, for example, writes:

> [. . .] in Meditation VI [Descartes] appealed explicitly to this principle [read: the causal principle according to which all the reality that exists in the idea objectively must be in its cause either formally or eminently] in support of [the] claim [that bodies cause sensory ideas]. He argued there that the cause of sensory ideas must formally or eminently contain what is contained objectively in these ideas. After affirming that it is inconsistent with the veracity of God that the cause of these ideas eminently contains this objective reality, Descartes concluded that bodies must cause the ideas [. . .]. He simply assumed that bodies formally contain what is contained objectively in sensory ideas.[37]

In a more recent article, Schmaltz discusses the passage from Meditation Six where Descartes writes: "[. . .] from the fact that I perceive by my senses a great variety of colours, sounds, smells and tastes [. . .] I am correct in inferring that the bodies which are the *sources* of these various sensory perceptions possess differences *corresponding* to them, though not resembling them" (CSM II 56; AT VII 81, emphasis added). According to Schmaltz, "this passage indicates that sensory ideas that do not resemble bodily qualities nonetheless are systematically correlated with them. *Because* of these correlations, particular ideas can direct the mind to certain bodily qualities rather than others."[38] The reasoning is that since the systematic correlation between the perception of colors (and the like) and bodies is due to the fact that the latter are the sources of the former, particular ideas "direct the mind to" (or represent) bodies because they are caused by them.

Other texts, where Descartes discusses the proof for the existence of material things, could be cited in support of the causal reading. Gassendi, in the Fifth Set of Objections, had objected that he found the claim that ideas of material things can be derived from the mind

[37] Schmaltz (1992), p. 45. Many other Descartes scholars have invoked the argument for the existence of material things to make the case that bodies are causes of sensory ideas. Daniel Garber, for example, writes: "The argument in Meditation VI clearly asserts that bodies have an 'active faculty' that corresponds to the 'passive faculty' of sensation; the clear implication is that the *body* that exists in the world is the cause of my sensation of it" (Garber (1993), pp. 19–24). However, insofar as Garber's arguments do not imply that the causal connection is responsible for the representationality of sensation, I will not discuss his views here.

[38] Schmaltz (2006), pp. 16–17; see also Schmaltz (1992), p.46.

bewildering (CSM II 204; AT VII 293). But Descartes, in the Fifth Set of Replies, denied that he had ever asserted that "ideas of material things are derived from the mind" (CSM II 253; AT VII 367). And he added: "Later on [i.e., in Meditation Six] I explicitly showed that these ideas often come to us from bodies, and that it is this that enables us to prove the existence of bodies" (Ibid.). A similar claim is made in a letter to Hyperaspistes dated August 1641 where Descartes writes that "[he] proved the existence of material things not from the fact that we have *ideas* of them but from the fact that these ideas come to us *in such a way as to make us aware that* they are not produced by ourselves but come from elsewhere [i.e., from material things]" (CSMK 193; AT III 429, emphasis added).

Let's pause for a moment and reflect upon these texts. Do they justify the causal theorists' claim that, according to Descartes, sensory ideas represent bodies because they are caused by them? I will provide four reasons in support of a negative answer. The first depends on arguments already developed in 3.5 above. As argued there, according to the causal principle, bodies are able to cause ideas of sense only *because* the properties of bodies are similar to the representational content of the ideas (since bodies contain formally the primary qualities of bodies that our ideas of sense contain objectively). But then the representational content of the idea must be available before, and independently of, a causal explanation on pain of circularity. And so, it must be the very *nature* of the representational content of sensory ideas that allows the causal explanation of their representational content rather than being the causal connection that explains the nature of the representational content of the ideas. Accordingly, the use of the causal principle in Meditation Six is still within the framework of Descartes' internalism.

The second reason relates to the first and goes back to Descartes' theory of ideas as outlined in Chapter 1. Descartes, in Meditation Three, claims that ideas of sense are like *images* of things because they *represent* things. Ideas represent things, along the lines of DA, by way of *presenting* an object to the mind. So, the causal principle, when applied to the objective reality of ideas, essentially implies that an object can be regarded as the cause of that idea only if it instantiates the properties described in its mode of presentation, that is, if it *satisfies* its description. But then the *description* of the object must be available before the causal principle is applied. Notice that this reading is in accord with the conclusion of the argument in Meditation Six. There, bodies are said to cause ideas of sense not because they are "similar" or "quasi-similar" to the sensory representation of them but because they satisfy the description of them according to the clear and distinct ideas of the intellect:

> God [. . .] has given me a great propensity to believe that [sensory ideas] are produced by corporeal things. So I do not see how God could be understood to be anything but a deceiver if the ideas were transmitted from a source other than corporeal things. It follows that corporeal things exist. They may not all exist in a way that exactly corresponds with my sensory grasp of them, for in many cases the grasp of the senses is very obscure and confused. *But at least they possess all the properties which I clearly and distinctly understand* [. . .]. (CSM II 55; AT VII 80, emphasis added)

Descartes writes that bodies are the causes of our sensory ideas because they instantiate all the properties that we would *clearly* and *distinctly* understand body to possess if we paid attention to the innate representation of body (latently present in our mind). Descartes infers that bodies are the causes of our sensory ideas because, according to the causal principle, bodies satisfy the intellectual description of the object of thought (latently and obscurely) contained in sensory ideas. This reasoning confirms that sensory ideas represent bodies in virtue of internal features of the ideas themselves rather than in virtue of a causal connection with bodies. And this conclusion is compatible with the use of the causal principle in the proof.

The first two reasons show that, if the causal principle proves anything about how the content of sensory ideas is determined, it proves exactly the opposite of what CA wants it to prove. But there is a third reason why the causal principle cannot do the work CA attributes to it. The principle was introduced in Meditation Three to prove whether *there exist* things (other than the mind) on the basis of the *ideas* we have of them; and in Meditation Six the principle is invoked to prove the *existence* of bodies.[39] Once this is clarified, the mistake of causal readings becomes apparent. Causal accounts like Schmaltz's misunderstand the

[39] This is confirmed by Axiom V in Descartes' Second Replies: "How do we know that the sky exists? [...] The only reason why we can use this idea as a basis for the judgment that the sky exists is that every idea must have a really existing cause of its objective reality; and in this case we judge that the cause is the sky itself. And we make similar judgments in each case" (CSM II 116–117; AT VII 165).

role of the causal principle within Descartes' philosophy. The role of this principle consists in inferring the *existence* of material things *on the basis of* how they are already (and non-relationally) represented rather than in explaining the *representational content* of the ideas. And so, causal accounts confuse the causal principle *qua* a tool to prove the existence of bodies on the basis of how they are (already) represented for a tool to explain the representationality of sensory ideas.

Finally, supporters of CA read the argument for the existence of material things as a metaphysical argument, i.e., as an argument based on how the content of sensory ideas is determined (that is, bodies must exist since the content of sensory ideas is determined by a causal connection with bodies). But aside from the difficulties mentioned above, the problem is that the argument in Meditation Six is an *epistemic* argument.[40] The argument begins with the assumption that we have sensory ideas and that these ideas represent or exhibit objects to us. According to Descartes, we know by the natural light that "in order for an idea to contain such and such objective reality, it must surely derive it from some cause which contains at least as much formal reality as there is objective reality in the idea" (CSM II 28–29; AT VII 41). So, sensory ideas need a cause. Descartes concludes that this cause is body (or corporeal nature) because we have "*a great propensity to believe that* [ideas of sense] are produced by corporeal things" (CSM II 55; AT VII 80) and, so, God would be a deceiver if they came from God rather than from corporeal things. Hence, corporeal things exist *qua* causes of our sensory ideas. Notice that this conclusion derives directly from the premise that we *believe* that ideas come from external things rather than directly from some premise about the representational content of sensory ideas. No doubt it is the representational content of the ideas (i.e., the fact that they exhibit bodies) that engenders this belief. Still, from the fact that the belief must be true on pain of God's being a deceiver it does not follow necessarily that *the causal connection* with bodies is what makes the ideas (that engender that belief) have the content they exhibit. The content could be determined in some other way and, as we have seen so far, there are good grounds to believe that this is in fact the case.

[40] I am indebted to Martha Bolton for urging me to think of the implications of this feature of the argument.

In light of the above reasons, I conclude that the argument for the existence of material things in Meditation Six leaves wide open the question of how the content of sensory ideas is determined. Accordingly, the proof is compatible with the internalist explanation of the representationality of sensation outlined in 5.2 above.

5.4 THE ROLE OF THE CAUSAL CONNECTION IN SENSORY REPRESENTATION: THE EVIDENCE FROM THE MIND–BODY UNION

Descartes unqualifiedly acknowledged that the causal interaction with bodily states plays some role in the production of sensory ideas. The texts are clear on this subject. Sensory perception is the product of the union of the mind with the body. Although "we know for certain that it is the soul which has sensory perceptions, and not the body" (CSM I 164; AT VI 109), it is also clear that, according to Descartes, these sensory perceptions are brought about either proximally by bodily states or distally by configurations of matter or by both (as it happens in normal circumstances in the case of the external senses).

In Meditation Six, Descartes clarifies that our nature *qua* the combination of mind and body (CSM II 57; AT VII 82) teaches us that "when I feel pain there is something wrong with the body" (CSM II 56; AT VII 80) and that when I have sensations of color and the like "various other bodies exist in the vicinity of my body" (CSM II 56; AT VII 81). Similarly, in Principles I.48, Descartes lists all sensations ("such as those of pain, pleasure, light, colours, smells, sounds, smells [. . .]", CSM I 209; AT VIIIA 23) as "certain [. . .] things" that we experience in ourselves (CSM I 209; AT VIIIA 23) and that arise from the union of our mind with the body. This point is repeated in the Sixth Set of Replies (CSM II 294; AT VII 437), in the correspondence with Princess Elizabeth (CSMK 218; AT III 665; CSMK 227; AT III 691–692) and in the *Passions of the Soul* (see for example, Part I.27, CSM I 338–339; AT XI 349).

The mechanisms by which sensations arise from the mind–body union are illustrated by Descartes in many passages from various philosophical and scientific works. Some texts suggest that different configurations of body and/or different motions in the brain *cause* sensations in us; other texts suggest that different bodily states *occasion*, or *provide a sign for*, the mind to form corresponding sensations; and other texts suggest that the relation between body and mind is instituted by nature. Here's a sample.[41]

The use of the causal principle in the proof for the existence of material things in Meditation Six and Descartes' use of the verb "producere" (CSM II 55; AT VII 79) when talking about the origin of ideas of sense suggest that these ideas are *caused* or *produced* by bodies. The same suggestion is in a letter to Elizabeth dated 21 May 1643, where Descartes claims that the body has the power to act on the soul and to "*cause* its sensations and passions" (CSMK 218; AT III 665).[42] And, in the *Passions of the Soul,* Descartes writes that our perceptions of external objects "are caused by these objects" (CSM I 337; AT XI 346).[43]

In the *Principles of Philosophy*, Descartes claims that various motions in the brain (originating in the external objects stimulating the sensory nerves) *affect* the mind in various ways (so as to elicit different sensations) or *excite* different sensations in the mind. For example:

> Sensory awareness comes about by means of the nerves, which stretch like threads from the brain to all the limbs, and are joined together in such a way that hardly any part of the human body can be touched without producing movement in several of the nerve-ends that are scattered around in that area. This movement is then transmitted to the other ends of the nerves which are all grouped together in the brain around the seat of the soul [. . .]. The result of these movements being set up in the brain by the nerves is that the soul or mind that is closely joined to the brain is *affected* in various ways, corresponding to the various different sorts of movements. (CSM I 280; AT VIIIA 316)[44]

In Principles IV.191, we are told that "external bodies possess what is required to bring it about that our nerves *excite* (*excitant*) in the soul the sensation of hardness, heaviness, heat, etc." (CSM I 282; AT VIIIA 318).

[41] For an insightful discussion of the various differences in the texts, see Wilson (1991).

[42] The French reads: "enfin, pour l'âme seule, nous s'avons que celle de leur union, de laquelle dépend celle de la force qu'a l'âme de mouvoir le corps, et le corps d'agir sur l'âme, en causant ses sentiments et ses passions."

[43] The French reads: "Celle que nous rapportons à des chose qui sont hors de nous, à savoir, aux objets de nos sens, son causées [...] par ces objets [...]."

[44] The Latin reads: "Motus autem qui sic in cerebro a nervis excitantur, animan sive mentem intime cerebro conjunctam diversimode *afficiunt*, prout ipsi sunt diversi" (AT VIIIA 316).

And, in Meditation Six, Descartes claims that "any given movement occurring in the part of the brain that immediately affects the mind [brings about] (*infert*) just one corresponding sensation" (CSM II 60; AT VII 87).[45] Similarly, in *Comments on a Certain Broadsheet*, Descartes employs an occasional language according to which corporeal motions "give the mind the occasion to form [ideas of secondary qualities] by means of a faculty innate to it" (CSM I 304; AT VIIIB 359).

Other texts tell us that the mind *is ordained by nature* to have certain sensations in correspondence with certain motions in the brain:

> [. . .] it is [motions in the brain] which, acting directly upon our soul in so far as it is united to our body, *are ordained by nature* to make it have such sensations. [. . .] [R]egarding light and colour [. . .] we must suppose our soul to be of such a nature that what makes it have the sensation of light is the force of the movements taking place in the regions of the brain where the optic nerve-fibres originate, and what makes it have the sensation of colour is the manner of these movements. (CSM I 167; AT VI 130, emphasis added)

Similarly, in the *Treatise on Man*, Descartes writes that when God unites a soul to the body "he will make its nature such that the soul will have different sensations corresponding to the different ways in which the entrances to the pores in the internal surface of the brain are opened by means of the nerves" (CSM I 102; AT XI 143).

In a few places, Descartes also writes as if the motions in the brain serve as *signs* for the mind to have certain sensations. In Meditation Six, Descartes writes that every time the part of the brain containing the common sense "is in a given state, it presents the same signals to the mind" (CSM II 60; AT VII 86); for example, "when the nerves in the foot are set in motion in a violent manner, this motion, by way of the spinal cord, reaches the inner parts of the brain, and there gives the mind its signal for having a certain sensation (*ibi menti signum dat ad aliquid sentiendum*), namely, the sensation of a pain as occurring in the foot" (CSM II 60; AT VII 88). But the most well-known passage where Descartes puts forward (what has been called) the "presentational model" is in the *Treatise on Light*:[46]

[45] My translation here is slightly different from Cottingham's. Cottingham translates "infert" as "produces" but that is not the exact sense of the Latin verb.

[46] The expression "presentational model" is from Wilson (1991).

[...] if words, which signify nothing except by human convention, suffice to make us think of things to which they bear no resemblance, then why could nature not also have established some sign which would make us have the sensation of light, even if the sign contained nothing in itself which is similar to the sensation? (CSM I 81; AT XI 4)

These passages offer the beginning of an answer to the question I asked at the end of section 5.2, *viz.*, what role *if any*, does the causal interaction with bodies play in Descartes' theory of sensory representation? The unifying theme in all these texts is that in having sensory experiences (unlike in the case of pure understanding) the mind is *affected* by different variations in bodies. Sensory ideas are not generated by the mind alone but in connection with the body insofar as different configurations of matter and motions in the brain affect the mind in different ways. And despite the *prima facie* textual differences, it is possible to interpret the way in which body affects the mind in *causal* terms. First, neither the heterogeneity doctrine nor the doctrine of the innateness of all ideas seems to rule out, for Descartes, the causal interaction between mind and body.[47] Second, the occasional, semantic

[47] The heterogeneity doctrine is supposed to rule out mind–body causal interaction (roughly) as follows. Since efficient causation requires some likeness between cause and effect and mind and body, according to Descartes, do not share any attribute, there cannot be any genuine causal interaction between mind and body. For this kind of argument see, for example, Broughton (1986) and Radner (1971) and more recently, Gorham (1999) and (2002). However, in a letter to Clerselier, Descartes writes that the problem of mind–body causal interaction "arises simply from a supposition that is false and cannot in any way be proved, namely that, if the soul and the body are two substances whose nature is different, this prevents them from being able to act on each other" (CSM II 275; AT IX A 213). For a defense of the possibility of mind–body causal interaction see Bedau (1986); Loeb (1981); O'Neill (1987); Richardson (1982); Rozemond (1999) and Schmaltz (1992). Moreover, causal interaction between mind and body is compatible with Descartes' view that ideas of sense are innate. Descartes himself often emphasizes that his nativism does not prevent him from maintaining that ideas become available to the subject on occasion with encounters with the environment. In *Comments on a Certain Broadsheet* Descartes clarifies that ideas are innate to us as certain diseases are innate to some families. As children of those families do not suffer from the disease in their mother's womb but are genetically disposed to contract it later in life, so too infants are not born possessing ideas but possessing dispositions to attain them later in life (CSM I 303–304; AT VIIIB 358). And, after claiming that external things "[...] transmit something which [...] gives the mind occasion to form [...] ideas [of secondary qualities]," Descartes insists that "[t]he ideas of pain, colours, sounds and the like [are] innate" (CSM I 304; AT VIIIB 359). It seems plausible to conclude that Descartes acknowledges that sensory ideas become available to us (or are acquired by us) on the

and institution-of-nature language of the above passages is *not* incompatible with the causal language of the first set of passages. When Descartes claims that different configurations of body or different brain states are ordained by nature to occasion, or provide a sign for, the mind to form some corresponding sensations Descartes may still regard the different configurations of body or brain states as remote *causes* of sensory ideas.[48] Occasional causation (to which both the institution of nature and presentational views may be reduced) is still a form of efficient causation. Configurations of matter are efficient causes of sensory ideas by way of providing the occasion for the mind to produce certain corresponding sensory ideas. It is also worth noting that acknowledging that body can (metaphysically speaking) act on the mind in the senses specified above does not undermine the conclusions of Chapter 3 and 5.3 above. For it is possible to acknowledge body-to-mind causation *without* accepting the view that the causal interaction explains why sensory ideas represent the kind of objects that they do. Whether different configurations of body are efficient, occasional or semantic causes, the causal connection with bodily configurations, in my view, is insufficient to explain why sensory ideas represent modes of *res extensa.*[49]

Since the above texts testify that a causal connection with bodies plays *a* role in the formation of sensory ideas; and since the arguments of Chapter 3 and 5.3 above establish that this role cannot consist in explaining why sensory ideas represent bodies, I conclude that the above passages indicate that, for Descartes, the causal connection with bodies accounts for the *phenomenal aspect* of sensory ideas. Although, no doubt, it is the mind that allows us to sense colors in general it is *only in virtue of the causal connection with bodies* that we experience, for example, the phenomenal red as opposed to the phenomenal green. The "substantial union" of mind and body and the causal connection between our mind and external bodies is what makes us have sensations

occasion of causal encounters with the environment. The question of the sense in which sensory ideas are innate remains an interesting one, but this is not a question that I will address here.

[48] For Descartes' distinction between proximate and remote causes see CSM I 305; AT VIIIB, 360. For the suggestion that bodily states could be partial causes of sensory ideas see Wilson (1991); Nadler (1994); O'Neill (1987) and Schmaltz (1992).

[49] Thanks to Daniel Garber for bringing this feature of my view to my attention.

of heat, color and so on. The mind *alone* cannot explain why we have the sensation of red as opposed to the sensation of green. Different bodies or different types of configurations of matter are the causes of different types of sensations or phenomenal appearance.

In Meditation Six, it is the explanation of the phenomenal aspect of sensory ideas that does not require any intellectual act and that is independent of the will. In Principles II.1, Descartes writes that "all our sensations undoubtedly come to us from something that is distinct from our mind (*quicquid sentimus, procul dubio nobis advenit a re aliqua, quae a mente nostra diversa est*). For, it is not in our power to make ourselves have *one sensation rather than another*"(CSM I 223; AT VIIIA 40, emphasis added). This aspect of Descartes' view on the production of sensory ideas has not received a proper degree of attention in the literature. Supporters of a purely internalist reading ignore it; and supporters of a causal reading mistakenly explain the intentionality of sensory ideas in virtue of the causal connection with bodies (as we saw in Chapter 3 above).

So, let me conclude with some remarks and questions that I will address in the following section. It is clear that, according to Descartes, the explanation of the *origin* of sensory ideas requires the postulation of a causal connection between the mind and the surrounding environment. But a theory of the origin of ideas is different from a theory of content determination. A causal connection with instances of x can be a necessary condition for the acquisition of the sensory idea of x but may have nothing to do with the explanation of why sensory ideas represent the kind of objects they do. So, should we conclude that the external relation with bodies plays *no* role whatsoever in the determination of the representational content of sensory ideas? In light of what I argued in Chapter 3 and in sections 5.2 and 5.3 above, this seems to be the right conclusion to draw. But this conclusion is hasty and partially inaccurate. Things are not so simple, at least in Descartes' case. I will argue that paying the right attention to the fact that, according to Descartes, the mind's causal interaction with bodies explains the phenomenal aspect of sensory ideas will clarify the sense in which the causal transaction with bodies still plays *some* role in the determination of the representational content of sensory ideas. Admitting this role will *not* commit Descartes to a causal theory of content but will *qualify* his internalism, at least in the case of sensory ideas. Accordingly, this admission is consistent with the conclusions of Chapter 3 and sections 5.2 and 5.3 above.

5.5 A DESCRIPTIVIST-CAUSAL ACCOUNT

In this section, first, I present what I call "a descriptivist-causal account." Then, I will explain the sense in which this account acknowledges that a causal connection with bodies still plays *some* role in the determination of the representational content of sensory ideas without falling into the pitfalls of causal accounts and while preserving (although qualifying) Descartes' internalism.

As we saw in Chapter 1, all ideas have both a presentational and referential content, according to Descartes. The referential content of the idea consists in the object of thought; its presentational content consists in the way in which the object of thought is presented to the mind. The presentational and referential contents constitute the representational properties of ideas. And along the lines of a descriptivist account of ideas (DA), the former determines the latter. However, according to Descartes, the object of thought can be presented to the mind in at least two different ways. It can be presented either obscurely and confusedly, as in the case of sensory ideas, by way of what I called "sensory presentational content;" or clearly and distinctly, as in the case of the clear and distinct ideas of the intellect, by way of what I called "intelligible presentational content." Whereas in the case of clear and distinct ideas, the idea of *n* cannot represent *n* as other than *n* is (since the description that identifies the object of thought is clear and distinct), in the case of ideas of sense the idea of *n* can indeed represent *n* as other than it is (since the idea represents its object as having some properties that in fact it does not have). So, to use an analogy, sensory ideas refer to their objects as other than they are in the same way in which a picture may be an inaccurate representation. Although the picture is the picture of the object being represented (because, say, it contains all the identifying properties of the object being represented) it may depict the object as having colors (or other properties) that the object does not actually have. Consequently, the picture represents the right object although it also contains a bunch of other features that obscure what the object is really like. That's why sensory ideas represent objects *as they appear to us* as opposed to as to how they really are. Only the intellect can provide us with the latter kind of representation. Accordingly, with sensory ideas, there *seems* to be a discrepancy between the presentational and referential content, that is, between the object as it is presented to us and the object as it really is. It is this feature of sensory ideas that has prompted some scholars to conclude that the referential content of sensory ideas is determined independently of the presentational content. I deny this conclusion and, so, I proceed to explain why sensory ideas exhibit this feature while preserving Descartes' overall commitment to DA.

Ideas of sense constitute a special class of ideas for they are the product of the substantial union of mind and body. As such, I argue, their *presentational content* is determined by two factors. On the one hand, as we saw in 5.4, the causal connection of the mind with external bodies accounts for why things in the world *appear to us* in a certain way. That is, it accounts for the phenomenology that accompanies any idea of sense. On the other hand, the *object* being presented to the mind is not determined by the causal connection (Chapter 3 and 5.3); rather it is determined by a latent conceptual description of the object (5.2). So, had Descartes been asked to explain the mechanisms that determine sensory content he would have said that these mechanisms combine causal and cognitive/descriptive factors as follows. On the one hand, the causal connection between different types of configurations of matter and the mind is what makes us have certain sensation types other than others on the occasion of different circumstances. It is a certain type of arrangement of particles on the surface of a body that makes me have the sensation of red rather than green. The mind alone cannot explain the difference in the phenomenology. On the other hand, the causal connection alone is insufficient to explain why the various sensations (so caused) are *about, or represent,* their causes. The mind must provide the conceptual resources not only for thinking of something external to the mind that causes the sensation (that is, the mind must provide a causal description such as "the object that is the cause of"), but also must enable us to conceptualize this object as such and such, that is, as an object that satisfies a certain identifying description (for example, as a body having the properties of extension and so on). As suggested at the end of Chapter 3 and explained more fully in section 5.2, this descriptive content is supplied by the innate ideas and principles of the mind. So, the presentational content of ideas of sense is determined by two factors because the (latent) conceptual description of the object coming from the mind is *naturally* (given the mind–body union) mixed with the phenomenology coming from the mind's interaction with the environment.

Even if the sensation-type is the product of the mind's causal interaction with different types of configurations of matter, it is the mind that refers the phenomenology to external objects. One may object that this explanation implies that judgment plays a role in the account of the representationality of sensation (when the mind refers the sensation Φ to x, the mind judges that x is Φ) and, hence, contradicts the arguments of Chapter 2 above. But this *prima facie* contradiction is easily dismissed. Any act of judgment, according to Descartes, is volitional in character.[50] But ideas of sense are independent of our will.[51] The *trompe l'oeil* violin painted on a door looks like a violin hanging on the door even if our intellect tells us that it is an illusion. We cannot help seeing it that way. We perceive red as a property of material objects even if the intellect tells us that material things have no qualitative properties. The stick partially submerged in water looks crooked even if we know that it is not. And so on. But if our sensory representations of the world were the product of a judgment and all judgments are volitional we should in principle be able to correct our sensory perceptions and see the external world the way it actually is. But we cannot and that's a strong indication that no judgment is involved in mechanisms of sensory representation. When Descartes speaks of *referring* our sensations to external objects,[52] he means that we perceive the redness and sweetness (that we feel) *as* a property of body or – *mutatis mutandis* – we experience bodies *as* red and sweet.[53] The representational content of ideas is then the product of a complex or structured perception rather than being the product of a judgment.[54] It is the product of the natural

[50] See, for example, CSM II 39–42; AT VII 56–61; CSM I 204; AT VIIIA 18 and CSM I 307; AT VIIIB 363.

[51] On this see, for example, CSM II 26; AT VII 38; and CSM II 55; AT VII 79.

[52] See, for example, *Passions of the Soul*, I.23, CSM I 337; AT XI 346. It is the fact that we cannot but perceive things this way that provides the best evidence for interpreting the "referring" language this way.

[53] The equivalence between saying "we perceive the redness and sweetness *as* a property of body" and saying "we perceive bodies *as* red and sweet" is important here because it implies a denial of the view that the mind takes pure sensations (or *qualia*) *as the primary objects of thought* and, then, attributes to them qualities that belong to the body.

[54] In this respect my views are similar to Brown (2006) although we disagree on what sensations represent and why they represent it. Deborah Brown persuasively argues that we should "compare the function of 'referring' in Descartes' epistemology to the notion of 'seeing as' in contemporary analyses of perception" (Brown (2006) pp. 100–101) and insists that "[o]ne advantage of the seeing-as talk over the talk of judgments is that it

union of the phenomenal aspect of sensory perception coming from the mind's causal interaction with the environment and the conceptualization of the cause/object of the sensation coming from the internal resources of the mind. Accordingly, when Descartes says that we refer the sensation of green to the grass he is saying that we perceive the grass as green or that we perceive greenness as a property of the grass rather than saying that we judge that the grass is green. We ought to keep the content of experience distinct from judgments based on that experience. My account honors this distinction.[55]

One may ask: why should we call this account "descriptive-*causal*" given that the object of ideas of sense is determined by the latent description provided by the innate conceptual apparatus? Why not simply say, along the lines of purely internalist accounts, that the occurrence of certain types of sensory ideas is regularly caused by the presence of certain types of bodies (or configurations of matter) but that this is the condition that satisfies their presentational content rather than what determines their content?[56]

Descartes' discussion of the etiology of sensation (see 5.4 above) makes clear that the causal connection is an integral part of a process that culminates with sensory representation. Even if it is the mind that conceptualizes the object of the idea of red as a body that causes the idea and, so, a description/conceptualization enters into the characterization of the causal connection, the causal connection is real. A causal connection that is cognitively processed is still a causal connection. Consequently, although the descriptive content carried by the sensory idea includes a causal connection between the idea and the object it refers to,

enables one to ascribe structured representational content to a perception without collapsing the distinction between perception and belief" (Ibid., p. 101). As I already indicated in 2.6 above, I agree with Brown on this.

[55] The suggestion has been made in the literature that the representational content of sensory ideas may be the result of non-volitional judgments (at least at the third grade of sensation). On this see, for example, Simmons (2003). According to Alison Simmons, non-volitional judgments "affect the way the world appears to us. They do not immediately result in any *beliefs* about the world but rather in a sensory *experience* of it" (Simmons (2003), p. 567). Since there is no obvious account of this kind of judgment in Descartes and since it is possible to explain the representationality of sensation in an alternative way which has more textual grounding, I prefer not to use the terminology of judgment at all when dealing with the account of the representationality of sensation. For a similar point see Brown (2006), p. 101 and 2.6 above.

[56] This objection was made to me by Martha Bolton in a private exchange.

the causal connection contributes something – i.e., the sensory appearance of the object – which is *not already* contained in the *mind's* description of the object of thought.

A proponent of a purely internalist account can still rejoin: since sensory ideas are regularly caused by their right objects *because this is the condition that satisfies the mind's way of presenting of the object of thought*, the causal connection has nothing to contribute to the explanation of *what* ideas of sense *represent*. The theory is purely descriptive. I will argue that there are at least two distinct (but related) contributions that the causal connection makes in the explanation of what sensory ideas represent.

First, notice that a theory of content ought to account for why an idea is an idea of x rather than of y. However, as the conclusion of the argument for the existence of material things in Meditation Six testifies (CSM II 55; AT VII 80), the mind can at most conceptualize the object of sensory ideas as some configuration of matter or other. The mind could at most only determine that the sensation S represents some type of configuration of matter or other. So, *some other factor needs* to complement the internalist story if we want to have a satisfactory account of what makes a sensation S represent one type of configuration of matter rather than another. It is from this potential impasse for an internalist theory that a causal account (CA) gains its (apparent) strength.[57] On CA, this problem does not arise. Ideas represent their right objects because they are caused by them in regular ways. Unfortunately, as we saw in Chapter 3, CA suffers from other serious difficulties and cannot be Descartes' considered position. But it is possible to have an overall internalist theory that incorporates a causal element. On this theory, *the (qualitatively) different ways in which the object of sensory ideas appears to us* by way of the causal connection with bodies is (at least) one of the factors that induce the mind to differentiate among the various objects (or causes) of sensory ideas. How? The causal connection between that type of configuration of matter and the mind contributes *something* (for example, the phenomenal appearance of red) that *together with* the mind's conceptualization of the object of thought (as some configuration of matter causing the idea) constitutes the presentational content that determines the object of ideas of sense (for example, a particular type of configuration of matter that resembles the felt sensation of redness). As we shall see later

[57] Thanks to Tad Schmaltz for emphasizing this point to me.

(5.7), these two aspects of the presentational content of sensory ideas are metaphysically inseparable. They are fused together in a seamless experience that makes the external world *appear* to us in certain (and erroneous, according to Descartes' physics) ways.

To summarize, the fact that sensory ideas represent particular types of configurations of matter depend on two factors. The different types of phenomenal states tell the mind that there are different types of configurations of matter that cause different ideas; but it is the mind that conceptualizes the object of thought as a configuration of matter that causes (or corresponds to) the idea. So, although the mind's sensory representation of bodies is the result of a cognitively mediated causal connection, the causal link between the mind and the environment still provides the mind with *empirical* cues to differentiate among different ideas and their objects. The causal connection alone could not fix the object of the idea without the mind's already representing the *kind* of object we are causally connected with; the mind alone would not be able to distinguish one body from another. Therefore, in so far as the phenomenal content of sensory ideas contributes to the individuation of their objects; and the mind's causal interaction with the environment accounts for this phenomenal content, the mind's causal interaction with the environment plays some role in Descartes' theory of sensory representation.[58]

This last consideration brings us to the second contribution of the causal connection in Descartes' account of sensory content. The manner in which bodies appear to us qualitatively reflects the mind's causal interaction with the environment. Since the manner in which bodies appear to us *qualitatively* is an integral part, and the distinguishing mark, of *sensory* representation, the mind's causal interaction with the environment contributes to the determination of the presentational

[58] In his comments on my "On Causal Accounts of the Representationality of Cartesian Sensations" at the meeting of the Eastern Division of the American Philosophical Association (December 27–30, 2007), Desmond Hogan suggested that Descartes' internalism *must* include contextual elements on pain of having the unwanted consequences of having two presentationally-identical ideas refer to the same thing. My idea of red, for example, refers to the red couch in my living room every time I am there and I look at it; but it refers to the red coat in my closet every time I open the closet and look at it. My above suggestion on how to qualify an internalist theory is compatible with Hogan's remark. The causal link provides the contextual cue, or determines the presentational context, that helps distinguish not only two ideas of red but also different types of sensory ideas (such as the idea of red and the idea of green).

content of sensory ideas as much as the (latent) conceptual description of the object of thought. More precisely, in the case of sensory ideas, the presentational content is obscure and confused. This obscurity and confusion (as we shall see in more detail in 5.7) is generated by the natural confusion of the qualitative aspect of sensation (coming from the mind's interaction with the environment) with the conceptual description of the object of thought. The phenomenal character of experience *and* the description of the object of thought *together* constitute the presentational content of sensory ideas. The former, so to speak, obscures the latter, hence yielding sensory ideas that represent their correct objects obscurely or as having some properties that they do not actually have. This is why the idea of red, for example, represents bodies as if they instantiated a property resembling the phenomenal red. But *this confused object of thought* (*viz.*, a mode of *res extensa* allegedly resembling the felt sensation as opposed to a mode of *res extensa* as it actually is) is the object of *sensory* representation. Since the presentational content that determines the object of sensory ideas is partly constituted by a phenomenal content deriving from the mind's causal interaction with external bodies, any account of Descartes' views on sensory representation that does not include the role played by the causal connection is bound to be incomplete.

For the above reasons, I conclude that Descartes' account of sensory representation is "descriptive-causal." I am well aware that the sense in which I call Descartes' account "causal" is different from modern-days causal theories of content. This is not surprising. Descartes' way of thinking of ideas is inconsistent with the possibility (that causal theories embrace) that an idea can stand for an object of which the subject is completely unaware. Wilson's remark that "the causal account was influential in Descartes' thought even if he was unable to develop it fully"[59] may be, after all, correct. But it needs qualification. My account shows the extent to which the causal account was influential in Descartes' thought (without committing him to an unlikely causal theory of content) and it explains why he was unable to develop it fully.[60]

[59] Wilson (1990), reprinted in Wilson (1999), p. 76.

[60] The term "descriptivist-causal" was coined by Sterelny (1983) and then used by Devitt and Sterelny (1987), in order to criticize purely causal theories of reference-fixing. Their criticism is that purely causal theories suffer from what they call the "qua-problem." For an

5.6 THE DIFFERENCES BETWEEN A DESCRIPTIVIST-CAUSAL AND PURELY INTERNALIST ACCOUNTS

The similarities between my descriptivist-causal account and internalist ones are apparent. But what distinguishes them? Does my account have any advantages over purely internalist ones? I will address these questions in this section, although the answers are already implicit in what I argued above.

As we saw in 5.1 above, Pessin's account (despite his claims to the contrary) provides *no* internalist account of the representationality of sensation. Pessin claims that sensations, like intellectual ideas, represent their objects in virtue of *internal* relations between the idea and the representandum. Intellectual ideas represent their objects internally because "Fred's direct [...] awareness of [his] thinking of the sun is just his (*cognitively*) direct awareness of the sun."[61] Given the analogy between intellectual and sensory ideas, one would expect Pessin to explain how "Fred's awareness of his sensing of yellow is his (*cognitively*) direct awareness of motion-m."[62] That is, one would expect Pessin to explain *in cognitive terms* the something internal to the sensation of yellow that makes it a representation of motion-m. However, no such explanation is forthcoming. Unable to explain why sensations (*cognitively*) intrinsically represent their objects *even if they are obscure and*

explanation of this problem see Chapter 3 above. Marga Reimer describes Devitt's and Sterelny's descriptive causal theory as a hybrid theory according to which a "descriptive element is needed to handle what Devitt calls the '*qua* problem'" and whose point is that in order to know "what kind of object one is naming [one has to] conceptualize that object, to think of it as an object of a certain sort, as [...] satisfying a certain predicate. It is thus to think of it *qua* such-and-such. Thus, if an act of reference-fixing is to be successful, the reference-fixer must think of the referent-to-be under a certain description – one that that object or individual 'fits'" (Reimer (2003)). I believe that Devitt's and Sterelny's general idea *helps* understand Descartes' view on sensory representation although I would not go as far as saying that their views are exactly the same as Descartes'. For one thing it is not clear to me in what sense the causal connection determines content, in Devitt and Sterelny's hybrid theory. But I am pretty sure that whatever this sense may be it is not the same as the one I attribute to Descartes.

[61] Pessin (2009), p. 10.
[62] Ibid., p. 10.

confused, he concludes that the representationality of sensations is not only intrinsic but a *primitive*. However, this conclusion is self-defeating since, in the end, *no* internalist account is provided.

A descriptivist-causal account provides the theoretical and textual resources to solve this difficulty in Pessin's view. Sensory ideas (intrinsically) represent their correct objects despite their obscurity because of the mind's latent conceptualization of the object of thought. Although we may not be directly aware of this conceptualization, the latter is latently contained in our sensory ideas (in so far as it determines the object or content of our sensory appearances). This latent intellectual content is what allows us to be *minimally* aware of the object of ideas of sense[63] and, hence, have minimal *epistemic access* to it.

As we saw above, my internalist explanation of the representationality of sensation takes inspiration from Bolton's account, although I develop it in ways Bolton did not originally intend.[64] But there are clear differences between our accounts. According to Bolton, the object of sensory ideas is *ultimately* fixed by the clear and distinct ideas of the intellect. However, insofar as she does not explain why these ideas initially seem to represent *qualities of bodies that resemble the felt sensation*; and *this is* the way in which *sensory* ideas represent their objects in normal circumstances, Bolton does not provide a satisfactory account of *sensory* representation proper. Moreover, Bolton seems to suggest that the mind has all the resources in itself to fully answer the question of why different ideas represent different types of bodies or different types of configuration of matter.[65] But how can the mind alone explain why different sensory ideas represent different types of configurations of matter? After all the intellectual understanding of the object of thought can only give us an understanding of the essential properties of matter and hence it would fail to distinguish one material object from another. A descriptivist-causal account solves these two difficulties by reintroducing a role for a causal element to play within an overall internalist account. The different types of phenomenal appearances that

[63] I borrow the expression "minimally aware of" from Bolton (1986).

[64] For example, I am not sure Bolton would agree with the way I relate Descartes' doctrine of simple notions with his theory of innate ideas. I read Descartes' claim that every thought contains simple notions that determine its intentional content as equivalent to the claim that some innate ideas are latently operative in our thoughts and structure them.

[65] Bolton has suggested this to me in a private exchange.

derive from the mind's causal interaction with bodies and that are constitutive of the presentational content of sensory ideas explain both why sensory ideas represent qualities of bodies that resemble the felt sensations and why different ideas of sense represent different bodies or configurations of matter.

I should add that Bolton (1986) suggests an explanation of why different sensory ideas end up representing different bodies:

> In Meditation Six, sense experience is considered as a whole [. . .]. When taken as elements in a more complex experience, perceptions of heat and the like have a representative character they lack when considered apart. In the context of an experience that represents bodies by other devices, striking phenomenal differences represent significant variations among bodies. But in order to play this role, ideas of heat, color and so on, do not need to be individual representations of bodies. It is critical to identify what the unit of representation is; it is not isolated ideas of color and heat, but a complex pattern in which these ideas are elements.[66]

According to Bolton, a holistic constraint makes the ideas of heat and red representative of different configurations of matter. Be this as it may, it is the causal connection that endows us with what she calls "striking phenomenal differences" and, so, the causal connection must be taken into account also.

For all these reasons, I conclude that my descriptivist-causal account of Cartesian sensations is to be preferred to currently available purely internalist ones.

5.7 THE PUZZLE OF SENSORY REPRESENTATION EXPLAINED

Ideas of sense, like all ideas, have both a presentational and referential content. The exegetical question is whether, in the case of sensory ideas, their referential content is determined by the presentational content (along the lines of DA) or independently of it (along the lines of externalist theories). Given that, according to Descartes, sensory ideas are misrepresentations of their objects, they must represent them. But, then, what theory of sensory representation would explain why Descartes maintains

[66] See Bolton (1986), p. 400.

that ideas represent their objects as other than they are *in normal circumstances*? Does Descartes hold a theory of sensory representation along the lines of DA? And if so, what kind of qualifications should be added to such a theory so that it accommodates cases of misrepresentation and avoid Arnauld-like objections? Or should we attribute to Descartes a completely different theory of sensory representation? Perhaps a causal theory? The *prima facie* advantage of causal theories consisted precisely in their explanation of sensory misrepresentation. On causal accounts, Descartes would claim that ideas of sense represent their correct objects as other than they are because what fixes the "correct" objects of sensory ideas is not the presentational content of these ideas but a causal connection. Accordingly, an idea can (referentially) represent its (correct) object although it may (presentationally) represent it as other than it is. But I established in Chapter 3 that causal theories fail to explain either why ideas of sense represent bodies in the first place or why they misrepresent them. On purely internalist accounts, such as Bolton's, an explanation is provided for why sensory ideas ultimately represent what they do (i.e., modes of *res extensa*) but there is no explanation of why they mis(re)present them. So, does a descriptivist-causal account fare any better in explaining sensory misrepresentation?

The answer is yes. This becomes clear if we highlight (a) the importance of Descartes' claim that all sensory ideas are *obscure and confused* representations; and (b) the fact that the presentational content of these ideas is determined by two inseparable factors, as suggested in 5.5 above. Descartes relates the notion of misrepresentation to that of obscurity and confusion in several places.[67] But what makes sensory ideas obscure and confused? On my account, sensory ideas are obscure and confused representations of their objects because they *embody* the fusion of the latent conceptualization of the object (coming from the mind) and a phenomenal content (coming from a causal connection with a particular type of configuration of matter). So, according to Descartes, on the one hand, sensory ideas *represent their objects* because

[67] See, for example, CSM II 30; AT VII 43–44 and CSM II 164; AT VII 234. One may object that when Descartes claims that sensory ideas are obscure and confused he means to say they lack an intentional object. If this is the case, my account is in trouble. But the very fact that Descartes calls sensations "ideas" (and all ideas are, by definition, representational, CSM II 25; AT VII 37) suggests that sensory ideas are obscure and confused in the sense that we cannot *fully* detect what their object is.

they *present* them correctly in virtue of the innate ideas of body and extension that are latently present in sensory experience; but, on the other hand, they represent their objects *as other than they are* because their "true" representation is obscured by the confusion with the phenomenal appearances coming from the causal connection with the environment. Accordingly, sensory ideas represent their objects as other than they are, along the lines of an internalist theory, because their presentational content contains not only the identifying description of the object of thought but also the associated qualitative aspect derived from the causal connection with the environment. A sensory idea mispresents its object because it contains a confused description of the right object of thought. A descriptivist-causal account can then explain cases of misrepresentations while avoiding Arnauld-like objections.

Let me explain further. As we saw in Chapters 1 and 2 the idea of red is the sensation *of* red where "of red" ought to be taken as an objective genitive (*viz.*, as "the sensation of something red outside the mind) as opposed to a subjective genitive (*viz.*, as "the sensation of redness itself"). This is so because, on my account, the presentational content of ideas of color encompasses two elements:

(i) A phenomenal content – *viz.*, the sensation of red as such or the phenomenal red.
(ii) A conceptualization of the object of thought as a property of body causing the sensation.

Notice that I draw this distinction between (i) and (ii) only for expository purposes and in order to illustrate the mechanism of misrepresentation. I do not mean to suggest that these two aspects of ideas of sense are distinct or exist separately from one another in the sensing mind, according to Descartes. On the contrary, as we saw in 5.5 above, the representationality is built-into the phenomenology of ideas of sense. The mind endowed with the innate ideas of body and so on is the same mind which, united with the body, experiences particular things. Consequently, it cannot but apply its categorial knowledge to what it experiences (be it the inner or the outer world). We can certainly focus attention on one aspect of the sensory idea in abstraction from the other, but neither aspect exists in the sensing mind without the other. In fact, confusing these two aspects (so that the mind cannot help but experience red as a property of bodies) explains why sensory ideas are intrinsically *confused* as opposed to being intrinsically *clear* but confused because of an implicit judgment we make. So, the idea of red does not have the sensation of red as its object; rather – given the way in which the presentational content of the idea is determined – the idea of red consists in our experiencing red as a property of body.[68]

Let's think again of the analogy with a picture and let's assume (in order to make the analogy work) that this picture represents its object by internal means rather than in virtue of external ones. Suppose that this picture is made by a blind artist who can nonetheless represent the essential properties of external objects by purely intellectual means.[69] According to Descartes, this picture would represent an external object as it actually is, that is, as something having the property of extension, shape and so on. Now suppose that this artist gains sight. His purely

[68] Beyssade (1992) seems to suggest something similar. He writes: "Our referring sense data to external objects [...] is not only a blind [...] impulse. All sensory qualities are connected with other qualities, the geometrical and mechanical qualities, which are given both to our senses and to our intellect. Now, figures and motions [are understood as if in objects.] And their connection with sensations is not a secondary act of judgment, which adds an *extra* objective reference to a mere internal affection, as learning a language adds an extra meaning to mere sounds. On the contrary, I am from the beginning aware of sensations of heat and cold [...] and *simultaneously* ideas of figure, motions and so on (whose represented content is easily perceived as things or modes of things). Therefore, the representational character of sensation meets a two-fold content: an internal psychological content (the subjective diversity of sense-data); and the objective represented content of geometrical ideas. [...] But the general representational character is supported by the *native* link between a non-representational content of various sensations and a represented content" (Beyssade (1992), p. 16, emphasis added). Despite the *prima facie* similarities, however, there is a clear difference between Beyssade's account and mine. Although according to Beyssade "the internal psychological content" never occurs in isolation from our perception of geometrical ideas, this internal content is *per se* non-representational ("[...] Descartes knew that all representational paintings ultimately involves non-representational [...] strokes" (Ibid. p. 18); "[materially false ideas are such that] I am unable to discriminate [...] whether or not there is some represented content in a sensation besides the affective psychological state itself" (p. 13)). This view amounts to denying that sensations are representational. Since it is by association with geometrical ideas that sensations gain representationality, the possibility that "[the geometrical ideas]' connection with sensations is [...] a secondary act of judgment, which adds an *extra* objective reference to a mere internal affection" is reintroduced, despite Beyssade's claims to the contrary. On my account, instead, the representationality is built-into the phenomenology so that there are no two things (the pure sensation and the idea) that occur together but one seamless perception, *viz.*, a sensory *idea*.

[69] Notice that this is a possibility that Descartes would allow since a blind person still possesses the idea of body.

intellectual representation of the external world would be blurred by the sensory appearances that now crowd his mind. These sensory appearances are the result of the newly gained causal connection of his mind with the environment. Let's also assume (given Descartes' view that the object of thought cannot be totally veiled from recognition) that these disturbances are not sufficient to blur his vision completely so that they do not prevent the artist from seeing bodies. However, these appearances would be enough to confuse the artist and cause him to believe that the world is actually colored or that the object being represented instantiates the sensible qualities of redness, greenness and so on. I want to say that, according to Descartes, we are in the same position as the artist who has gained sight. Our ideas of sense are intrinsically confused and it is their intrinsically confused presentational content that leads us to make erroneous judgments about the world.[70]

Let me now provide textual evidence that the natural confusion of these two aspects of ideas of sense is the source of sensory misrepresentation. In the Fourth Set of Replies, Descartes explains that ideas of color and the like are "more" materially false than others as follows:

[70] Kurt Smith makes the similar suggestion that sensations are complex modes that include a representational component. See Smith (2005), pp. 569–570. Accordingly, for example, the idea of red *presents* redness although it *represents* some motions of particles (Ibid., especially pp. 579–583). However, our views are radically different for at least two reasons. First, according to Smith the representational component of the sensation is to be explained in causal terms (Ibid., pp. 579–580, 574–575 and 581). Second, according to Smith, sensations *per se* are not representational although they contain a representational component. Sensations simply consist in our perceiving bluely or greenly. The argument by which Smith establishes that a sensation, although it carries an ideational component, is not itself an idea, is as follows: "[...] although the sensation has [...] as one of its constituents an idea, which is representational by nature, the sensation qua modal complex is not representational. This is not difficult to understand. If Jones, for instance, were to give to Smith a photograph of the Empire State Building, even though this act (of giving) includes in its description something that is representational, the fact that the photograph is representational does not transfer to the act of giving" (Ibid., p. 570). Likewise, the fact that a sensation has an idea as its constituent does not make the sensation representational. But notice that this "argument" is based on the (mistaken, according to me) assumption that the photo (idea) represents by means that are independent of the sensation experienced by the subject, that is, in virtue of a simple causal connection. In this case, there is a distinction between the sensation and the idea. But, on my view, the subject that is having the sensation is also the subject who contributes the conceptualization of the object of thought and so there is no real distinction between the sensation and the idea. There is only one thing, the sensory idea. The object of thought is not (totally) opaque to the sensing subject.

[. . .] ideas which give the judgment little or no scope for error do not seem as much entitled to be called materially false as those which give great scope for error. It is easy to show by means of examples that some ideas provide much greater scope for error than others. Confused ideas which are made at will by the mind, such as the ideas of false gods, do not provide as much scope for error as the confused ideas arriving from the senses, such as the ideas of color and cold. (CSM II 163; AT VII 233–234)

Descartes claims here that ideas of color and so on are "more" materially false than ideas of false Gods because the latter are confused complex ideas made up at will by the imagination whereas the former are *naturally* confused ideas. This claim is compatible with my claims that (i) sensory ideas are structured perceptions that embody the confusion of a conceptual and phenomenal element; (ii) that this confusion is the source of misrepresentation; and (iii) that this feature of ideas of sense is a product of the mind's natural union with the body.

In Principles I.45, Descartes defines clear and distinct perception as follows:

I call a perception "clear" when it is present and accessible to the attentive mind – just as we say that we see something clearly when it is present to the eye's gaze and stimulates it with a sufficient degree of strength and accessibility. I call a perception "distinct" if, as well as being clear, *it is so sharply separated from all other perceptions that it contains within itself only what is clear.* (CSM I 207–208; AT VIIIA 22, emphasis added)

An idea is clear when it is accessible to the mind with a certain degree of strength and *distinct* when we are able to keep the clear elements of the idea separate from other perceptions so as to avoid confusion (and, hence, to be able to identify the object of thought). By contrast, then, an idea is confused when we are not able to distinguish its clear elements from other perceptions. Accordingly, in my view, ideas of color (for example) are confused precisely because they are constituted by the fusion (or con-fusion) of the phenomenal and conceptual components. As such they are *intrinsically* confused representations, *viz.*, representations of their objects as other than they are.

But in Principles I.46, Descartes seems to suggest something different:

For example, when someone feels an intense pain, the perception he has of it is indeed very clear, but is not always distinct. For people commonly confuse this perception with an obscure judgment they make concerning the nature of something which they think exists in the painful spot and which they suppose to resemble the sensation of pain; but in fact it is the sensation alone that they perceive clearly. Hence a perception can be clear without being distinct [. . .]. (CSM I 208; AT VIIIA 22)

Descartes seems to deny here that sensations are intrinsic misrepresentations of their objects, as he himself claims in the *Meditations* and Fourth Set of Replies and as I interpret him. For in the above passage he writes that sensations alone (i.e., pure sensations) are clear and that their confusion (i.e., the fact that they represent their objects as other than they are) is the result of a mistaken judgment.[71]

This reading of the above passage is too simplistic. First, in Principles I.69, Descartes goes back to saying that our perception of color is *not as clear* as our perception of size and shape (CSM I 218; AT VIIIA 34). Second, as I argued in Chapter 2, I believe that it would not even be possible to make an erroneous judgment about nature of body unless we already experienced color as if it were a property of body. The intrinsic representationality of sensation is, so to speak, a necessary middle step. The very proof of the existence of material things in Meditation Six confirms this. Unless ideas of sense seemed to present bodies to us, we would have no reason to believe that they come from bodies and so the very grounds of the proof would be undermined. Third, we should consider the broader context of Principles I.46. Descartes is here discussing the genesis of our erroneous judgments and is telling us that it is possible to avoid them by distinguishing "the clear elements from those which are obscure or liable to lead us into error" (CSM I 208; AT VIIIA 22). And in the case of sensations, Descartes writes in Principles I.66, we avoid error, that is, we *clearly* perceive sensations, "provided that we take great *care in our judgments concerning them to include* no more than what is strictly contained in our perception – no more than that of which we have inner awareness" (CSM I 216; AT VIIIA 32).[72] Notice that here

[71] See Nelson (1996) on this. Also thanks to Steven Bayne for reinforcing the necessity to explain this passage in a way that is compatible with my account and Descartes' own former views.

[72] The title of Principles I.68 also suggests the same: "How to distinguish what we *clearly* know in such matters from what can lead us astray" (CSM I 217; AT VIIIA 33, emphasis added).

Descartes is saying exactly the opposite of what he says in Principles I.46 because he writes that the *clear* perception of color and pain is *the result of a judgment* (that, in turn, is based on our knowledge that bodies do not formally contain colors) rather than being its *original* status.[73] And we ought to read Principles I.46 in light of Principles I.66 and some of the following sections as follows. Once we acknowledge that ideas of sense are intrinsically confused and may lead us to err about the nature of the object that they represent, we can simply focus on the phenomenological aspect of the sensory ideas alone so as to avoid error. This is confirmed by Principles I.70 where Descartes describes two different ways of making judgments about the things perceived by the senses. On the basis of our perception of "colors in objects" (CSM I 218; AT VIII A 34), writes Descartes, we can either "merely judge that there is in the objects something [. . .] whose nature we do not know [. . .]" (Ibid.) "but which produces in us a certain very clear and vivid sensation which

[73] Tom Vinci has pointed out to me that Descartes may have been simply careless in Principles I.66 and the title (and some parts of) of Principles I.68. In light of what Descartes had claimed in Principles I.46 (that is, that a sensation can be clear without being distinct due to an erroneous judgment); and what he claims in Principles I.68 (that is, that "[i]n order to distinguish what is clear in this connection from what is obscure, we must be very careful to note that pain and colour and so on are *clearly and distinctly* perceived when they are regarded merely as sensations or thoughts" (CSM I 217; AT VIIIA 33)), according to Vinci, Descartes ought to have said, in Principles I.66, that sensations are *clearly and distinctly* perceived "provided that we take great care in our judgments concerning them to include no more than what is strictly contained in our perception – no more than that of which we have inner awareness." On this see Vinci (1998), pp. 198–203. If Vinci were right, then Descartes' view would be that the *distinctness* (rather than the clarity) of sensation would be the result of a judgment. And so, *contra* my view, color perceptions, would be intrinsically clear and pure sensations. But even if Vinci were right and Descartes expressed himself ineptly in Principles I.66 and 68, I don't believe Principles I.46 supports the view that, according to Descartes, color perceptions are devoid of any representational content and, hence, are intrinsically clear. Principles I.68 unequivocally tells us that color and the like are *regarded* merely as pure sensations as a result of a judgment. This implies that no matter how seemingly clearly they are perceived originally (as Principles I.46 tells us) they are not experienced by us as pure sensations. In fact, we can certainly experience pain very clearly even if we experience it *as if* in the foot. This reading is consistent with what Descartes wishes to argue in Principles I.46, that is, that the clarity of the perception has nothing to do with its distinctness. But it is only in virtue of a judgment (based on our knowledge that bodies do not formally contain colors) that we clearly and distinctly understand colors to be merely sensations that do not resemble anything in the material world. In conclusion, no matter how one reads Principles I.46, nothing in there supports the view that we experience color initially as a pure sensation devoid of representational content.

we call the sensation of colour" (Ibid.) – and in this case we would avoid error; or we could make the erroneous judgment that "what is called color in objects is something exactly like the colour of which we have sensory awareness" (Ibid.). What emerges clearly from Principles I.70 is that according to Descartes the error and confusion does not derive from a judgment that would turn the intrinsically clear idea into a confused representational one (as Principles I.46 seems to suggest). The error consists in *letting oneself being led into error* by the intrinsically confused content of the idea (that contains only a partially correct representation of the object). Accordingly, sensations are clearly understood when "in our judgments regarding them" we include no more than what we have inner awareness of or the "sensation alone." This would allow us to avoid error. So, even Principles I.46 is compatible with what Descartes maintains in the *Meditations* and Fourth Set of Replies. According to Descartes, sensory ideas are intrinsically confused and obscure ideas because they fuse together the representation of body (coming from the mind) with the phenomenal appearance (coming from a causal connection with bodies). Such fusion generates an obscure idea because the idea *represents body as colored.*

CONCLUSION

In this chapter, I presented my reading of Descartes' account of the representationality of sensation, *viz.*, what I called a "descriptivist-causal account." I explained the extent to which it shares important similarities with currently available internalist accounts but also why it differs from them. Then, I concluded with an explanation of how my account answers our exegetical question better than any other currently available theory. The exegetical question was: what theory of sensory representation should we attribute to Descartes that would explain why he maintains that ideas represent their objects as other than they are in normal circumstances? A descriptivist-causal account attributes to Descartes a theory of sensory representation along the lines of DA (and, hence, avoids the pitfalls of externalist readings) but qualifies it in ways that make it possible for it to explain the phenomenon of sensory misrepresentation while avoiding Arnauld-like objections (*viz.*, how can a Cartesian idea misrepresent in the sense of presenting one object to the mind but representing another?). As long as my account attributes to Descartes the view that sensory ideas are obscure descriptions of their *correct* objects, Arnauld-like objections are avoided and the mechanisms of sensory misrepresentation explained within an internalist framework.

6

Objections and Replies

In this last chapter, I address some possible objections to various aspects of my descriptivist-causal account. This will afford me the opportunity to further clarify my view.

6.1 ARE CARTESIAN *QUALIA* REINTRODUCED?[1]

In section 5.5 above, I argued that ideas of sense are misrepresentations because they embody a confusion of two aspects of content, i.e., the (intellectual) representation of body and phenomenal content. However, one may object that this view reintroduces through the back door the previously shunned reading of Cartesian sensations as *qualia.* If the intellectual representation of body needs to be added to the raw sensation in order to make it representative, the objection goes, then my view implies that sensations (like paint on canvas or mere sounds) do not represent anything by themselves. By combination with something else the *sensation itself* does not acquire the property of representationality.

This objection results from misunderstanding my account since it assumes that what I call the "fusion" of the representational and phenomenal content is a case of *addition* and, in so doing, it simply begs the question with me. The reasoning is that *since* sensations are devoid of representational content, they can only become representational either by adding to them a representational idea or by carrying a representational

[1] This objection was first brought to my attention by Richard Field in all its variations. I am very grateful to Field for all the challenging and helpful remarks he raised in the course of an intense correspondence we had on various aspect of my views. In private exchanges, Thomas Vinci and Laura Keating also made similar objections.

content;[2] but neither the adding nor the carrying would be enough to make sensations themselves representational. Notice that the implication of this reasoning is that the object of sensory perceptions is determined independently of the sensation, *viz.*, only by the pure idea of the intellect. But on my account, in perceiving colors, the sensation (or phenomenal content) is a *constitutive* part of how the object of thought is represented and that's precisely why it is so difficult to avoid making erroneous judgments on the basis of sensory perceptions.

Moreover, if what I call the "fusion" of the representational and phenomenal contents were a case of addition, the idea of red would turn out to be exactly the same as the ideas of a golden mountain and of a corporeal God. That is, it would be an idea put together at will by us and whose constituent components are really separable from one another. However, in the Fourth Set of Replies, Descartes insists that sensations of color and so on differ from other materially false ideas such as the ideas of a golden mountain and of a corporeal God. The former are *more* materially false than the latter because unlike the latter they are not made up at will by us (CSM II 163; AT VII 233–234). Certainly, the fact that sensations of color and the like are not put together by us at will does not necessarily imply that they are not compound ideas. But this conclusion would still not tell us anything about the nature of this compound. If we think of the compound as a whole whose "parts" can only be *thought of* independently of one another, the fact that sensations of color are structured perceptions does not imply that they are composed of two separable parts (the pure sensation and the representative idea).[3]

[2] The latter is what Smith (2005) proposes. However, it is not clear how a sensation is supposed to *carry* an idea.

[3] Thomas Vinci also claims that "our mature sensory experience is of a phenomenological *fusion* of colors and primary qualities" (Vinci (1998), p. 132, my emphasis) and that "the 'fused' form of sense experience [...] is the feature [...] that provides the 'material for error' of which Descartes speaks in Meditation III" (Ibid., p. 133). However, according to Vinci, this fusion is itself the result of an immature referral judgment, that is, a judgment made at a very early stage by children who "initially experience the world of physical objects as not phenomenologically fused with [...] sensations of color, heat and so on" (Ibid., p. 134). The best evidence for attributing this view to Descartes is, according to Vinci, Principles I.71. In contrast with Vinci, my view is that the infantile mind *starts with* the fused form of sense experience – what Vinci calls sensations in extensional form (Ibid., p. 133). Accordingly, I provide a different reading of Principles I.71 below. On my account, ideas of primary qualities *shape* the way we

In conclusion, the unity of representational and phenomenal content in sensory ideas ought not to be regarded as a case of addition of otherwise distinct and separable features. That's what I tried to convey by saying that the representationality is built-into, or ingrained in, the phenomenology. The point is that, according to Descartes, our cognitive apparatus is so constituted that there are no *pure* sensations. A pure sensation is the result of focusing on one aspect of a sensory idea in abstraction from the other, rather than being a separable component of the idea.

Richard Field has proposed a way of explaining how the intellect makes sensations representative while preserving the intuition that sensations *per se* are not representational. He argued that *the intellect* takes the pure sensation to represent a mode of *res extensa.*[4] Accordingly, the difference between my view and Field's would consist in the difference between claiming (respectively) that *the idea of the intellect structures the sensory appearance in a way that makes it of something* and claiming that *the idea of the intellect takes the non-representational sensation for something that the idea of the intellect represents.*

According to Field, we ought to distinguish sensations and ideas of sense. Sensations are non-representational modes of the mind. Ideas of sense are ideas of the intellect that take sensations as modes of *res extensa.* This interpretation, according to Field, is textually grounded in Descartes' Fourth Set of Replies, where Descartes would make clear that the mode that is objectively represented in the idea of cold is *not* a mode of *res extensa* (like I maintain) but a mode of the mind, i.e., a sensation. Here's the passage from the Fourth Set of Replies:

> When my critic says that the idea of cold "is coldness itself in so far as it exists objectively in the intellect," I think we need to make a distinction. For it often happens in the case of obscure and confused ideas – and the ideas of heat and cold fall into this category – that an idea is referred to something other than that of which it is in fact the idea. Thus if cold is simply an absence, the idea of cold is not coldness itself as it exists objectively in the intellect, but something else, which I erroneously mistake for this absence, namely a sensation which in fact has no existence outside the intellect. (CSM II 163; AT VII 233)

experience colors, taste and so on and that's why Descartes says that we *feel* colors *as if they* were in objects and *feel* pain *as if it were* in the body (CSM I 337; AT XI 347).

[4] See Field (1993).

According to Field, here Descartes claims that the ideas of cold and the sensation of cold are distinct. The idea of cold is "an idea that includes [the] sensation [of cold] as part of its objective content and represents it confusedly as being of the same nature as [. . .] a possible mode of matter."[5] Field does admit that the above passage is ambiguous between two different readings. The alternative reading is this: the idea of cold does not represent the sensation of cold; rather *it is* the sensation of cold. But "of cold" is to be taken as an objective genitive, that is, as meaning that we experience cold as a property of bodies. In this case, as Field puts it, "it is the sensation that objectively represents the sensible quality of cold as a mode of external bodies, albeit confusedly."[6]

Since Field acknowledges that the passage from the Fourth Set of Replies isn't conclusive, he cites as further evidence for his view that sensations aren't representational (and hence ought to be kept distinct from ideas of sense) Descartes' discussion of the piece of wax in Meditation Two and the distinction of the three degrees of sensation in the Sixth Set of Replies. I argued, in Chapter 2, that nothing in the Sixth Replies clearly indicates that, according to Descartes, the second degree of sensation has to do with non-representational sensations.[7] As to Descartes' discussion of the piece of wax in Meditation Two, I disagree that it proves that, according to Descartes, the senses do not represent bodies. According to Field, Descartes' conclusion that knowledge of the wax is obtained only through the intellect implies that, as Descartes also writes in the Second Replies, "bodies are not strictly speaking perceived by the senses at all" (CSM II 95; AT VII 132). However, the discussion of our knowledge of the piece of wax hardly confirms this conclusion. Descartes' point is that knowledge of the true essence of bodies is not given by the senses. But this conclusion does not even begin to imply that the senses fail to represent bodies to us. In fact, the senses are quite explicitly said to perceive bodies, even if obscurely and confusedly, in the following passage from Meditation Two:

> [. . .] the perception of [the true nature of the wax] is a case not of vision or touch or imagination – nor has it ever been, despite previous appearances – but of purely

[5] Ibid., p. 324.
[6] Ibid., p. 324. For a discussion of this passage from the Fourth Set of Replies (and Field's interpretation of it), see also 2.4 above.
[7] See 2.3 above.

mental scrutiny; and this can be imperfect and confused, as it was before [qua *sensory* perception], or clear and distinct as it is now depending on how carefully I concentrate on what the wax consists in. (CSM II 21; AT VII 31)[8]

But there is a different way of couching the original objection – one that helps to uncover the true nature of my disagreement with non-representationalist accounts. One may argue I am mistaking the psychological process by which, in early childhood, we come to confuse the clear idea of matter with sensations with the issue of the metaphysical status of sensations and representative ideas. One may acknowledge that Descartes' view is that in early childhood we confuse the clear idea of body with the various sensations *in judging* that there are colored objects around us. This confusion is a result of our bad judgments and, hence, it is only a psychological matter. But sensations and representative ideas are metaphysically distinct insofar as the former is non-representational.[9]

However, as I have clarified in different places in the book, my view is that, according to Descartes, *metaphysically speaking* sensations and representations aren't distinct – that is, they do not exist in the infantile mind as distinct perceptions. Sensory ideas *are* confused modes of thought constituted by a representational and phenomenal component. It is the metaphysics of sensory ideas that prompts us to make the erroneous judgments of early childhood rather than being these judgments that explain the confusion of sensory ideas.

One may insist that my view must be wrong in light of Principles I.71. At the beginning of Principles I.71, Descartes writes that in early childhood the mind was aware of pleasure and pains and "it did not refer these thoughts to anything outside itself" (CSM I 218; AT VIIIA 35); moreover, the mind was also aware of sensations of tastes, smells,

[8] For my reading of Meditation Two see 5.2 above. Besides, I find Field's conclusion that the idea of cold "is an idea of the intellect that represents a sensation as a possible corporeal mode" (Field (1993), p. 329) problematic in its own right. Sensations are modes of the mind–body union, according to Descartes; and, as such, they are something that the mind–body union *experiences* as opposed to being something that the mind represents through its intellectual ideas.

[9] Both Richard Field and Thomas Vinci have phrased the objection this way on separate occasions. Vinci, for example, in a recent correspondence, has commented: "[...] [c]olors *can* be attributed to the things that are referenced by the ideas of primary qualities in ordinary perceptual experience [...]. What does not work is the assignment of a doctrine of sensory representation to Descartes where sensations have intrinsic referential capacity."

sounds that "do not represent anything located outside our thought" (Ibid.). These claims, argues the proponent of Cartesian *qualia*, suggest that Descartes' view is that in early childhood we experience sensations as non-representational states of the mind. "At the same time," Descartes continues, "the mind perceives sizes, shapes, motions and so on, which are presented to it not as sensations but as things, or modes of things [. . .] *although it was not yet aware of the difference between things and sensations*" (Ibid., emphasis added). Then later on, as we start moving about, we become aware of the existence of particular bodies and the mind "attributes to [bodies] not only sizes, shapes, motions and the like, which it perceived as things or modes of things, but also tastes, smells and so on" (Ibid.). Accordingly, the mind judges that bodies not only have sizes and shapes but they also have colors and so on. But then, *contra* my account, the erroneous judgment is *not* based on a *primitive* confusion of the representational and phenomenal content because Descartes *distinguishes* between sensations and representative ideas at the beginning of Principles I.71. So, at best, the confusion is not a case of "fusion" but of confused *addition* of two otherwise distinct notions. Accordingly, the original objection stands.

I disagree with this reading of Principles I.71. At the beginning of Principles I.70 Descartes writes that we perceive "*colours in objects*" (rather than as properties of our own experience) and that "as long as we merely judge that there is in the objects [. . .] something whose nature we do not know, then we avoid error" (CSM I 218; AT VIIIA 34). I take this to mean that if we limit ourselves to judge from the confused representation of color that there is *something* in bodies that corresponds to our sensation, we would avoid error. Descartes continues:

> Of course, we do not really know what it is that we are calling a colour; and we cannot find any intelligible resemblance between the colour which we suppose to be in objects and that which we experience in sensation. But this is not something we do take account of; and *what is more*, there are many other features, such as size, shape and number which we clearly perceive to be actually or at least possibly present in bodies *in a way exactly corresponding to* our sensory perception or understanding. And so we easily follow into the error of judging that what is called colour in objects is *something exactly like the* colour of which we have sensory awareness. (CSM I 218; AT VIIIA 34–35, emphasis added)

Descartes is saying that besides ideas of color and the like we also have ideas of size, shape and so on. And he explains that since the latter ideas represent properties of things that exactly correspond to the way we experience them we make the mistake – by confusion – of also believing that our ideas of color represent properties that exactly correspond to the way we experience them. *But notice that the confusion is not between non-representational sensations and representative ideas but between representations that correspond exactly to their objects (since bodies instantiate the properties represented by the ideas, i.e., size and shape) and representations that do not exactly correspond to their objects (since bodies do not instantiate any property that resembles the felt sensation).*

This is what Descartes is repeating at the beginning of Principles I.71. First, when Descartes writes that in early childhood the mind experiences pains and pleasures, he also claims that we experience them as something happening to the body ("In our early childhood the mind was so closely tied to the body that it had no leisure for any thoughts except those by means of which it had sensory awareness of what was happening to the body" (CSM I 218; AT VIIIA 35)). Secondly, when Descartes writes that the mind also experiences sensations of color, taste and so on and that these sensations "do not represent anything located outside our thought" he may be simply repeating what he said in Principles I.70, that is, that these ideas do not represent anything outside our thought that resembles the sensation. But as pains and pleasures are attributed to something external to the mind (that is, our body) so colors and tastes are also attributed to something external to the mind (that is, bodies). In fact, I take Descartes to mean exactly this when he writes in Principles I.71, that "the mind is not yet aware of the difference between things and sensations" (CSM I 219; AT VIIIA 35). The mind is not yet aware of the difference between things and sensation precisely because it experiences sensations as if of things.

For all the above reasons, I conclude that the objection, in all its different versions, fails to establish that my descriptivist-causal account reintroduces *qualia*. I suspect that this kind of objection confuses the metaphysics of sensation in ordinary sensory experience with the metaphysics of sensation after "the intellect has examined the matter" (CSM II 57; AT VII 82). Ultimately, nobody denies that Descartes wants to say that "pain and colour [. . .] are clearly and distinctly perceived when they are regarded merely as sensations or thoughts" (CSM I 217; AT

VIIIA 33). This is a *judgment* that the mind makes *after* the intellect has revealed the true nature of matter. But from the fact that we can avoid making erroneous judgments about the properties of the material world by focusing only on what we have inner awareness of when we perceive, for example, the color red, it does not follow that for Descartes sensations exist originally in the mind as pure non-representational states. We should not mistake Descartes' claim that our erroneous judgments about the corporeal world can be corrected by keeping separate in our minds the two aspects of our confused sensory representations for Descartes' *explanation* of why we make these erroneous judgments – that is, because there are two separate perceptions in the mind that *we* confuse in sensory experience. In fact, Descartes' own claim that avoiding these errors is extremely difficult implies that sensations are not experienced by the mind as purely qualitative states.

6.2 IS THE "BIFURCATION READING" REINTRODUCED?

Alison Simmons argues against what she dubs the "bifurcation reading" of Descartes' account of the perception of primary and secondary qualities.[10] According to this reading, Descartes draws a wedge between the *pure sensing* of secondary qualities and *the intellectual perception* of primary qualities. Whereas our experience of secondary qualities pertains to the sensory faculty alone, experience of primary qualities involves the use of the intellect. The primary textual evidence offered in support of this reading is Descartes' distinction of the three degrees of sensation in the Sixth Set of Replies. The first degree has to do with the physiology of sensation. The second degree "comprises all the immediate effects produced in the mind as a result of its being united with a bodily organ which is affected in this way. Such effects include the perceptions of pain, pleasures, thirst, hunger, colours, sounds, taste, smell, heat, cold and the like, which arise from the union [. . .] of mind and body [. . .]" (CSM II 294–295; AT VII 437). The third grade

[10] See Simmons (2003). Simmons attributes this reading to, for example, Atherton (1990), pp. 19–22 and pp. 30–33; Jolley (1990), p. 92; Maull (1980); Secada (2000), chapters four and five; and Wilson (1992).

concerns the judgments we make about external things and the "calculation about the size, shape and distance" (CSM II 295; AT VII 437) of external things "that depends solely on the intellect" (CSM II 295; AT VII 438). The claims that the second degree of sensation pertains to perception of secondary qualities and that nothing more than this perception "should be referred to the sensory faculty" (CSM II 295; AT VII 437) *together with the claim* that the third degree of sensation involves judgment, the perception of primary qualities and the intellect have provided support for the bifurcation reading.

Simmons denies that Descartes held this view.[11] According to Simmons, Descartes drew a wedge "between sensory perception and purely intellectual perception"[12] rather than between the *pure sensation of secondary qualities* and the *intellectual perception of primary qualities.* On Simmons's view, "the intellect [. . .] operates in roughly the same way in our sensory experience of both primary and secondary qualities: *it alters the sensory image without in any way intellectualizing it.*"[13] "[. . .] [T]hrough third-grade judgments, the intellect adds details to our imagistic, sensory representation of these qualities."[14]

It has been suggested to me that my account of Cartesian sensory misrepresentation is an instance of the bifurcation reading insofar as it implies that sensory experience consists in the mixing of the clear and distinct intellectual representation of primary qualities and the purely sensory (or non-representational) perception of secondary qualities.[15] However, exactly the opposite is the case. My view counts as evidence *against* a "bifurcation theory" because it acknowledges a way of *representing* the corporeal world that it is *proper* to the senses (and, hence, distinct from the purely intellectual understanding of it) and in which the intellect plays a role *without* intellectualizing our sensory experience of the external world. I will show this in two different, but complementary, ways.

First of all, in Chapter 2, I argued that there are both textual and theoretical reasons for believing (*contra* the above reading of the passage

[11] For a similar view see Vinci (1998), pp. 116–122.
[12] Simmons (2003), p. 549.
[13] Ibid., p. 551. Emphasis added. For the same point see Vinci (1998), pp. 125–131.
[14] Ibid., p. 575.
[15] Thanks to Sean Greenberg for this point.

from Descartes' Sixth Set of Replies) that in the second degree of sensation colors and tastes are experienced as if "in objects" or "in space." Clearly then, I do not attribute to Descartes, as the proponents of the bifurcation reading are alleged to do, the view that the *sensory* perception of secondary qualities is non-representational. The second degree of sensation involves some perception of primary qualities in so far as the perception of color, for example, is articulated spatially. The question is: How do we explain the fact that color perceptions are representational or articulated spatially? According to the bifurcation theory, since at the second level of sensation there is no mention of primary qualities and these qualities are mentioned only at the third grade where the intellect and judgment are also mentioned, representation of space is tied up with the ideas of intellect and the faculty of judgment. However, as I argued in Chapter 2, this reasoning is inconclusive. Descartes' claim that the calculation of the size and shape of an object is the result of a judgment (or reasoning that involves the use of "some natural geometry") does *not* necessarily imply that the second level of sensation consists only in the non-representational perception of secondary qualities. It is possible that the sensation of color represents color as a property of bodies or as an extended expanse of color independently of any reasoning or implicit judgment. Then, in section 5.5 above, I fleshed out this claim. I argued that the innate ideas of body and its categorial features (with which the intellect is endowed, according to Descartes) are actively employed even in sensory perception of secondary qualities. This employment, however, does not consist in an act of (implicit) judgment or reasoning. Rather, the latent presence in our mind of the idea of body and its categorial features makes us visually *experience* redness *as* an extended expanse of color or *as* a property of extended bodies. So, the latent presence of these ideas is what explains, or structures, the content of our sensory experiences *on the basis of which* we make subsequent judgments about the external world.

One may object, however, that the spatial articulation of the sensation of color, at the second level of sensation, is independent of any intellectual element at all (whether or not that intellectual element implies judgment). Descartes, at the second level of sensation, would be talking about the *sensory or imagistic* apprehension of the world. That is, he would be talking about visual *sensations or images* of bounded color patches. And, as one may put it, it is certainly possible to see a triangular patch of color without a mathematical understanding of the property of the triangle.[16] The explanation of the representationality of sensation at the second level is also the main point of disagreement between Simmons (2003) and myself. Simmons suggests that the spatial articulation of our perception of secondary qualities depends only on the faculty of sensory perception and imagination.[17] I do not dispute the fact that, according to Descartes, sensory perception and imagination, unlike the pure understanding, make use of images. There is plenty of evidence that Descartes maintains this.[18] But I dispute the claim that the *representationality* of our sensations of secondary qualities depends only on the faculty of sensory perception and imagination. Notice that Simmons herself, as we saw in Chapter 4, provides a different account of the representationality of sensations in Simmons (1999). But the main problem is textual. Descartes suggests in several places that the images in the brain are not sufficient to explain why the mind (not the pure mind, but the mind as united with the body) represents what it does. In the *Optics*, Descartes writes that "[i]t is obvious that we judge shape by the knowledge or opinion that we have of the position of the various parts of an object, and *not by the resemblance of the pictures in our eyes.* For these pictures usually contain only ovals and rhombuses when they make us *see* circles and squares" (CSM I 172; AT VI 140–141).

After having criticized the Scholastic theory of sensory perception according to which "in order to have sensory perceptions, the soul must contemplate certain images transmitted by objects to the brain" (CSM I 165; AT VII 112), Descartes adds:

And if, in order to depart as little as possible from accepted views, we prefer to maintain that the objects which we perceive by the senses really send images of

[16] Tad Schmaltz has emphasized this difference to me in a private exchange.

[17] See Simmons (2003) especially pp. 559–563. On p. 562, for example, she writes: "[...] the spatial information represented in the retinal images and pineal inclinations has to get into the mind in the form of a second-grade sensations for it to play any role in our sensory experience at all." And on p. 572, Simmons writes: "To the extent that these constructive judgments are based on spatial qualities [...] they are based on sensory *images* of these qualities (either images stored in memory or images present at the second grade of sensory perception)," original emphasis. Again on p. 565: "Descartes [...] maintains that both imagination and sensory perception are distinctly imagistic modes of representation."

[18] See, for example, CSM II 51; AT VII 73; and CSM II 265; AT VII 387.

> themselves to the inside of our brain, we must at least observe that in no case does an image have to resemble the object it represents in all respects. It is enough that the image resembles its object in a few respects. [. . .]. You can see this in the case of engravings: consisting simply of a little ink placed here and there on a piece of paper, they represent to us forests, towns, people [. . .]; and although they make us think of countless different qualities in these objects, it is only in respect to shape that there is any real resemblance. And *even this resemblance is very imperfect*, since engravings represent to us bodies of varying relief and depth on a surface which is entirely flat. Moreover, in accordance with the rules of perspective they often represent circles by ovals better than by other circles [. . .] and similarly for other shapes. Thus it happens that in order to be more perfect as an image and in order to represent an object better, an engraving ought not to resemble it. Now we must think of the images formed in our brain in just the same way, and note that the problem is to know *simply how they can enable the soul to have sensory perceptions* of all the various qualities of the objects to which they correspond. (CSM I 165–166; AT VI 112–113, emphasis added)

Descartes suggests that a brain image is insufficient to explain why we see things the way we do *even if* brain images carry some spatial information. Besides, in a famous passage from his exchange with Gassendi, Descartes claims that although it is certainly possible to have visual representation of a triangular patch of color without having a mathematical understanding of the properties of the triangle, it is not possible to experience the patch of color *as* triangular unless the mind already possessed the idea of triangle.[19]

The second reason why my view is not an instance of the bifurcation reading can be found in section 5.2. I explained there why the mind cannot but perceive colors *as if they were properties of bodies.* I argued that because of the way in which the Cartesian mind is constituted (or endowed with the innate ideas of body and its categorial features), it naturally experiences red and cold *as properties of body* – *contra* the bifurcation reading. Accordingly, in my view, the intellect structures (and is active in) sensory experience without, as Simmons puts it, "*intellectualiz[ing]* the sensory representation."[20] Employment of these innate ideas (which are in the mind or intellect) does not amount to any

[19] See CSM II 262; AT VII 382; and also CSM I 212; AT VIII A 28.
[20] Simmons (2003), p. 574.

intellectualization of sensory experience since the representation of the external world is still in the form of a *sensory* – and potentially misleading (because obscure and confused) – representation. Sensing the world through our conceptual apparatus is still different from a purely intellectual understanding of it.

In conclusion, my claim that the intellect is active in our sensory apprehension of the external world does not amount to the claim that the intellectual clear and distinct ideas of body and its categorial features are mixed up with *pure* sensation. Rather it amounts to the claim that there is *no* pure sensation. And, so, since I believe that, according to Descartes, the innate ideas of the mind structure the phenomenological appearance of the world I do not attribute the bifurcation reading to him.

Contra the original objection, then, my account turns out to be a criticism of the bifurcation reading that shares some similarities with Simmons (2003). It differs from it, though, in one important respect. According to my reading, the intellect that structures the phenomenological appearance of the world is the same intellect that is endowed with innate ideas. According to Simmons, the intellect that structures the appearances of the world is the intellect "conceived quite generally as a faculty of perception and representation"[21] or is the "mind's ability to [. . .] represent things to itself."[22] Consequently, according to Simmons, Descartes' *distinction* between the sensory and purely intellectual representation of the world implies that the two are completely independent of each other (sensory representation, be it at the second or third level of sensation, is never based on the intellectual ideas of primary qualities). According to my reading, Descartes does distinguish between sensory representation (which is obscure and confused) and intellectual representation (which is clear and distinct) but the former is dependent on the latter (while preserving its *sensory* nature). Despite this disagreement, however, Simmons and I agree that Descartes drew a wedge between sensory representation and purely intellectual representation rather than between the pure sensing of secondary qualities and the intellectual representation of primary qualities.

[21] Simmons (2003), p. 569.
[22] Ibid., p. 569.

6.3 WHY NOT A SEMANTIC-CAUSAL, RATHER THAN A DESCRIPTIVIST-CAUSAL, ACCOUNT?

According to a natural signification theory, Cartesian sensations represent (or refer to) external objects because, being regularly caused by these objects, they function as *natural signs* of them. This explanation avoids invoking any internalist element in the explanation of the representationality of sensations and employs, instead, the notion of natural sign to complement the causal account. Accordingly, some external event (say, a certain type of arrangement of particles on the surface of an object) causes a type of motion in the brain; this motion is a natural sign for the mind to produce correlated ideas that, in turn, signify or represent the states of the world that regularly cause them (i.e., the motions and ideas). This natural signification theory is also known as the "semantic model."[23] As words simply signify things rather than representing them because they fail to resemble them; so, sensations simply signify external bodies instead of representing them because they fail to resemble them.

The textual support for this reading comes primarily from the following passage from the *Treatise on Light*:

> [. . .] if words, which signify nothing except by human convention, suffice to make us think of things to which they bear no resemblance, then why could nature not also have established some sign which would make us have the sensation of light, even if the sign contained nothing in itself which is similar to the sensation? (CSM I 81; AT XI 4)

And, in Meditation Six, Descartes writes that sensations "*signify* nothing [of the essence of things located outside of us] that is not very obscure and confused (*corporum extra nos positorum essentia, de qua tamen nihil nisi valde obscure and confuse significant*)" (CSM II 58;

[23] See Yolton (1984). Recently, Andrew Chignell has defended a similar view and dubbed it "the semantic-causation model." See Chignell (2009). In an earlier version of the paper, Chignell maintained that brain states function both as signs for the mind to generate ideas and as signs of the objects that the ideas represent. However, in Chignell (2009), Chignell does not take a stand on whether sensations represent any object at all. As a result, some of the following objections to the natural signification theory will not apply to Chignell (2009).

AT VII 83).[24] This passage suggests that sensations are mere signs of the objects they refer to and, hence, that, contrary to my view, they do not contain any mode of presentation of the object being represented.

Despite this textual evidence, I disagree with a semantic reading of Cartesian sensations for several reasons. First, as we saw in previous chapters, there are several passages where Descartes classifies sensations among "ideas." One may object that sensations *cannot* be ideas because they fail to resemble their objects and, so, they cannot represent them. But this objection makes the mistaken assumption that resemblance is a necessary condition for representation. And, as is clear from Chapter 1, I believe that the representation relation for Descartes has nothing to do with resemblance. Ideas represent their objects by expressing some satisfaction conditions or an identifying description of their referent. So, even if sensations do not resemble their objects they could still contain (although obscurely and confusedly) some identifying description of their objects and represent them in virtue of such latent description. In fact, this is exactly what I think is the case, as we saw in Chapter 5.

Second, there is at least one passage where Descartes explicitly rejects the view that the mind *looks at* the images in the brain in order to form correlated ideas. In the *Optics*, Descartes writes:

> [W]e must not think that it is by means of [. . .] resemblance that [the image in the brain] causes our sensory perception of these objects – *as if there were yet other eyes within our brain with which we could perceive it.* Instead we must hold that it is the movement composing this picture which, acting directly upon our soul in so far as it is united to our body, are ordained by nature to make it have such sensations. (CSM I 167; AT VI 130)

This evidence, as many commentators have pointed out, should be sufficient evidence to discredit the semantic model.[25]

[24] My translation here differs from Cottingham's and it was inspired by Martha Bolton's translation of this passage (see Bolton (1986), p. 399). See also CSM II 59–60; AT VII 86–88.

[25] See, for example, Hatfield (2003), p. 242 and pp. 307–310; Wilson (1991), reprinted in Wilson (1999), pp. 52–57; and Simmons (2003), p. 561 and fn. 28 on p. 561. For an alternative reading of this passage that could block this kind of objection see Vinci (2005), pp. 54–55. Vinci's point is that it is possible to read the above passage from the *Optics* as disparaging the view that "the brain, not the soul, has another set of eyes" (Ibid., p. 55).

Third, and most importantly, the natural signification model presupposes the very notion of representationality that it is invoked to explain and, so, it lacks explanatory power. Descartes is explicit that the patterns in the brain need not resemble what causes them (CSM I 165–167; AT VI 112–131); so, it is not resemblance between the brain patterns and their causes that accounts for why the former are signs for the mind to produce ideas that represent the distal causes of the brain patterns. An explanation of how this happens is in order. In virtue of what is the mind capable of taking the brain patterns as signs to form ideas that end up representing the causes of these brain patterns (i.e., external bodies)? The brain pattern may cause the mind to have an idea that (in virtue of some already encoded representational content) represents its cause but does not explain why the mind is capable of producing that representational content. This capacity must come from internal resources of the mind. So, it is the mind's internal resources for representation that explain why we take brain patterns as signs to form certain ideas rather than being the signification relation that explains why our sensory ideas represent what they do. That is, brain patterns are taken as signs of their causes *because* of the ideas already provided by the mind (as my account confirms) rather than the other way around (as the semantic model claims). So, a semantic account is self-defeating since the notion of the mind's interpreting the brain states as signs requires the very representational abilities that the semantic account is intended to explain.[26]

[26] The seeds of this criticism can be found (if I read Hatfield correctly) in Hatfield (2003), p. 309.

Conclusion

The book provides a systematic account of Descartes' views on sensations of color and the like that not only establishes that Cartesian sensations are representational but also culminates with a new proposal of how to explain their representationality. One of the main advantages of this new proposal – what I called a "descriptivist-causal account" – consists in providing an adequate solution to the puzzle of sensory misrepresentation within Descartes' internalist theory of ideas while, at the same time, avoiding Arnauld-like objections.

Causal accounts misinterpret both the role that, according to Descartes, the causal interaction with bodies plays in the formation of ideas of sense; and the texts where this causal role is discussed (see especially 5.3 and 5.4). Moreover, as we saw in Chapter 3, causal accounts fail to explain both why sensory ideas are representations of their causes and the phenomenon of sensory misrepresentation.

Teleofunctional accounts mistakenly saddle Descartes with an unlikely teleofunctional theory of sensory *representation* on the basis of his attribution of a teleology to sensations. Besides arguing, in Chapter 4, that a teleofunctional account introduces several theoretical problems, I claim that it is possible to interpret the teleological jargon of Meditation Six in a way that abstains from attributing to Descartes a teleofunctional theory of representation. On my account, the causal connection explains the phenomenal aspect of sensory ideas. But, as it is clear from Descartes' discussion of the dropsy and phantom limb cases in Meditation Six, a benevolent God has not only preordained things in the world so that different types of sensations are caused by different types of configurations of matter that correspond to these sensations; but he has also correlated with different configurations of matter *the sensations (or phenomenal contents)* that are most conducive to the survival of the mind–body union (CSM II 60–61; AT VII 88). So, on my account, the causal connection with bodies together with the teleology of sensory ideas explains (at best) the phenomenal aspect of sensory ideas. All Descartes is saying is that God has ordained things so that ideas of sense (that represent bodies on independent grounds) represent bodies *in a way that* depends on the causal interaction with particular bodies and is conducive to the preservation of the mind–body union. Accordingly, the teleology at best explains why the objects of ideas of sense *are presented in a certain way* rather than explaining why the ideas represent these objects.

Current purely internalist accounts, I argued in Chapter 5, either fail to provide any account of the representationality of sensation or, if they do provide such an account, they fail to distinguish it from intellectual representation. I am sympathetic to internalist interpretations and I explain why at the end of Chapter 3 and in Chapter 5 (see especially 5.2). But I also reintroduce a role for the causal connection to play in Descartes' account of sensory representation and explain what this role is (see especially 5.5) This reintroduction allows my descriptivist-causal account not only to provide an adequate explanation of *sensory* representation (as opposed to intellectual representation) within Descartes' internalist theory of ideas (5.5–5.6) but also to solve the puzzle of sensory misrepresentation (5.7).

References

Adams, R. (1975). "Where do our Ideas Come From – Descartes vs Locke." In S. P. Stich (ed.), *Innate Ideas.* Berkeley, University of California Press, pp. 71–87.

Alanen, L. (1994). "Sensory Ideas, Objective Reality, and Material Falsity." In J. Cottingham (ed.), *Reason, Will and Sensation: Studies in Descartes' Metaphysics.* New York, Clarendon Press, pp. 229–250.

—— (2003). *Descartes's Concept of Mind.* Cambridge, Massachusetts, Harvard University Press.

Atherton, M. (1990). *Berkeley's Revolution in Vision.* Ithaca, Cornell University Press.

Ayers, M. R. (1991). *Locke. Epistemology and Ontology.* London, Routledge.

Bedau, M. (1986). "Cartesian Interaction." *Midwest Studies in Philosophy* 10, pp. 483–502.

Beyssade, J. M. (1992). "Descartes on Material Falsity." In P. D. Cummins and G. Zoeller (eds.), *Minds, Ideas and Objects: Essays on the Theory of Representation in Modern Philosophy.* Atascadero, Ridgeview, pp. 5–20.

Block, N. (1994). "Qualia." In S. Guttenplan, (ed.), *A Companion to Philosophy of Mind.* Oxford, Blackwell, pp. 514–520.

—— (2003). "Mental Paint." In M. Hahn and B. Ramberg (eds.), *Reflections and Replies: Essays on the Philosophy of Tyler Burge.* Cambridge, Massachusetts, MIT Press, pp. 165–201.

Bolton, M. (1986). "Confused and Obscure Ideas of Sense." In A. O. Rorty (ed.), *Essays on Descartes' Meditations.* Berkeley, University of California Press, pp. 389–404.

—— (1998). "Universals, Essences, and Abstract Entities." In D. Garber and M. Ayers (eds.), *The Cambridge History of the Seventeenth Century Philosophy,* 2 volumes. Cambridge, Cambridge University Press, pp. 178–211.

—— (2002). "La obra de Margaret Wilson." In L. Benitez and J. A. Robles (eds.), *Homenaje a Margaret Wilson.* México, DR, Universidad Nacional Autonóma de México, pp. 33–54.

Broughton, J. (1986). "Adequate Causes and Natural Change in Descartes' Philosophy." In A. Donagan, A Petrovich and M. Wedin (eds.), *Human Nature and Human Knowledge.* Dordrecht, Reidel, pp. 107–128.

Brown, D. (2006). *Descartes and the Passionate Mind.* Cambridge, Cambridge University Press.

Chappell, V. (1986). "The Theory of Ideas." In A. O. Rorty (ed.), *Essays on Descartes' Meditations*. Berkeley, University of California Press, pp. 177–198.

—— (1997). "Descartes' Ontology." *Topoi*, 16, pp. 111–127.

Chignell, A. (2009). "Descartes on Body–Mind Relations: The Semantic-Causation Model." *Philosophers' Imprint*, 9, 5, pp. 1–22.

Clarke, D. (1982). *Descartes' Philosophy of Science*. Manchester, Manchester University Press.

Cook, M. (1987). "Descartes' Alleged Representationalism." *History of Philosophy Quarterly*, 4, pp. 179–195.

Cottingham, J. (1986). *Descartes*. Oxford, Blackwell.

Crane, T. (2001). *Elements of Mind*. Oxford, Oxford University Press.

Dennett, D. (1988). "Quining Qualia." In D. J. Chalmers (ed.), *Philosophy of Mind*. Oxford, Oxford University Press, pp. 226–246.

De Rosa, R. (2004). "Descartes on Sensory Misrepresentation: the Case of Materially False Ideas." *History of Philosophy Quarterly*, 21, 3, pp. 261–280.

—— (2004a). "The Question-Begging Status of Locke's Anti-Nativist Arguments." *Philosophy and Phenomenological Research*, 69, 1, pp. 37–64.

—— (2008). "Review of Cecilia Wee's *Material Falsity and Error in Descartes's Meditations*." *Journal of the History of Philosophy*, 46, 4, pp. 641–642.

—— and Bueno, O. (2008). "Descartes on Mathematical Essences." *Protosociology. An International Journal of Interdisciplinary Research*, 25, pp. 160–180. The volume is also published by Ontos Verlag http://www.ontos-verlag.de/Buchreihen-LOGOS-978-3-86838-009-5.php.

Descartes, R. (1964–1974). *Oeuvres de Descartes*. Ed. C. Adam and P. Tannery, vols. I–XI. Paris, Libraire Philosophique J. Vrin.

—— (1984–1985). *The Philosophical Writings of Descartes*. Ed. and trans. J. Cottingham, R. Stoothoff and D. Murdoch, Volumes I–II. Cambridge, Cambridge University Press.

—— (1991). *The Philosophical Writings of Descartes. The Correspondence*. Ed. and trans. J. Cottingham, R. Stoothoff and D. Murdoch, Volume III. Cambridge, Cambridge University Press.

Devitt, M. and Sterelny, K. (1987). *Language and Reality*. Cambridge, Massachusetts, MIT Press.

Field, R. (1993). "Descartes on the Material Falsity of Ideas." *The Philosophical Review*, 102, 3, pp. 309–333.

Fodor, J. (1987). *Psychosemantics*. Cambridge, Massachusetts, MIT Press.

—— (1990). *A Theory of Content and Other Essays*. Cambridge, Massachusetts, MIT Press.

Frankfurt, H. (1970). *Demons, Dreamers, and Madmen*. Indianapolis, Bobbs-Merrill.

Garber, D. (1993). "Descartes and Occasionalism." In S. Nadler (ed.), *Causation in Early Modern Philosophy.* University Park, Penn State University Press, pp. 9–26.

Gorham, G. (1999). "Causation and Similarity." In R. Gennaro and C. Huenemann (eds.), *New Essays on the Rationalists.* Oxford, Oxford University Press, pp. 296–309.

—— (2002). "Descartes on the Innateness of All Ideas." *Canadian Journal of Philosophy,* 32, pp. 355–388.

Greenberg, S. (2007). "Descartes on the Passions: Function, Representation, and Motivation." *Nous,* XLI, pp. 714–735.

Grene, M. (1985). *Descartes.* Minneapolis, University of Minnesota Press.

Gueroult, M. (1985). *Descartes Philosophy Interpreted According to the Order of Reasons.* Volume II. Edited and translated by Roger Ariew. Minneapolis, University of Minnesota Press.

Hatfield, G. (1998). "The Cognitive Faculties." In M. Ayers and D. Garber (eds.), *Cambridge History of Seventeenth Century Philosophy.* Cambridge, Cambridge University Press, pp. 953–1002.

—— (2003). *Descartes and the Meditations.* London and New York, Routledge.

Hoffman, P. (1996). "Descartes on Misrepresentation." *Journal of the History of Philosophy,* 34, pp. 357–381.

Jolley, N. (1990). *The Light of the Soul: Theories of Ideas in Leibniz, Malebranche, and Descartes.* Oxford, Oxford University Press.

Kendrick, N. (2000). "Why Cartesian Ideas of Sense are Innate." *The Southern Journal of Philosophy,* 38, pp. 413–428.

Kenny, A. (1968). *Descartes: A Study of His Philosophy.* New York, Random House.

Kripke, S. (1972). *Naming and Necessity.* Cambridge, Massachussetts, Harvard University Press.

Loar, B. (2003). "Transparent Experience and the Availability of Qualia." In Q. Smith and A. Jokic (eds.), *Consciousness.* Oxford, Clarendon Press, pp. 77–96.

Leibniz, G. W. (1996). *New Essays on Human Understanding.* Ed. and trans. P. Remnant and J. Bennett. Cambridge, Cambridge University Press.

Loeb, L. (1981). *From Descartes to Hume: Continental Metaphysics and the Development of Modern Philosophy.* Ithaca. Cornell University Press.

MacKenzie, A. W. (1990). "Descartes on Sensory Representation: A Study of the Dioptrics." *Canadian Journal of Philosophy,* Supplementary Volume 19, pp. 109–147.

Malebranche, N. (1997). *The Search After Truth.* Ed. and trans. T. M. Lennon and P. J. Olscamp. Cambridge, Cambridge University Press.

Maull, N. (1980). "Cartesian Optics and the Geometrization of Nature." In S. Gaukroger (ed.), *Descartes: Philosophy, Mathematics and Physics.* Sussex, Harvester Press, pp. 23–40.

McRae, R. (1972). "Innate Ideas." In R. J. Butler (ed.), *Cartesian Studies.* Oxford, Basil Blackwell, pp. 32–54.

Nadler, S. (1989). *Arnauld and the Cartesian Philosophy of Ideas.* Manchester University Press, Manchester, 1989.

—— (1992). *Malebranche and Ideas.* Oxford, Oxford University Press.

—— (1994). "Descastes and Occasional Causation." *British Journal for the History of Philosophy,* 2, pp. 35 –54.

Nelson, A. (1996). "The Falsity in Sensory Ideas: Descartes and Arnauld." In E. J. Kremer (ed.), *Interpreting Arnauld.* Toronto, University of Toronto Press, pp. 13–32.

Nolan, L. (1997). "The Ontological Status of Cartesian Natures." *Pacific Philosophical Quarterly,* 78, pp. 169–194.

—— (1998). "Descartes' Theory of Universals." *Philosophical Studies,* 89, pp. 161–180.

Normore, C. (1986). "Meaning and Objective Being: Descartes and his Sources." In A. O. Rorty (ed.), *Essays on Descartes' Meditations.* Berkeley, University of California Press, pp. 223–241.

O'Neill, E. (1987). "Mind–Body Interaction and Metaphysical Consistency: A Defense of Descartes." *Journal of the History of Philosophy,* 23, pp. 227–248.

Peacocke, C. (1983). *Sense and Content: Experience, Thought, and Their Relations.* Oxford, Oxford University Press.

Pessin, A. (2009). "Mental Transparency, Direct Sensation, and the Unity of the Cartesian Mind." In J. Miller (ed.), *Topics in Early Modern Philosophy of Mind,* forthcoming, Springer, pp. 1–37.

Radner, D. (1971). "Descartes' Notion of the Union of Mind and Body." *Journal of the History of Philosophy,* 9, 1971, pp. 159–170.

Reimer, M. (2003). "Reference." In *Stanford Encyclopedia of Philosophy.* http://plato.stanford.edu/entries/reference.

Richard, M. (1997). "Propositional Attitudes." In B. Hale and C. Wright (eds.), *A Companion to the Philosophy of Language.* Oxford, Blackwell.

Richardson, R. C. (1982). "The 'Scandal' of Cartesian Interactionism." *Mind,* 92, pp. 20–37.

Rodis-Lewis, G. (1990). *L'Anthropologie Cartesienne.* Paris, Presses Universitaires de France.

Rorty, A. (1986). "Cartesian Passions and the Union of Mind and Body." In A. O. Rorty (ed.), *Essays on Descartes' Meditations.* Berkeley, University of California Press, pp. 514–534.

Rozemond, M. (1999). "Descartes on Mind–Body Interaction: What is the Problem?" *Journal of the History of Philosophy,* 37, 3, pp. 435–467.

—— (2008). "Descartes' Ontology of the Eternal Truths." In P. Hoffman, D. Owen and G. Yaffe (eds.), *Contemporary Perspectives on Early Modern*

Philosophy: Essays in Honor of Vere Chappell, forthcoming, Broadview Press, pp. 41–63.

Schmaltz, T. M. (1992). "Sensation, Occasionalism and Descartes' Causal Principle." In P. D. Cummins and G. Zoeller (eds.), *Minds, Ideas and Objects: Essays on the Theory of Representation in Modern Philosophy*. North American Kant Society Studies in Philosophy, Atascadero, Ridgeview, pp. 37–55.

Schmaltz, T. M. (1997). "Descartes on Innate Ideas, Sensation, and Scholasticism: the Response to Regius." In M. A. Stewart (ed.), *Oxford Studies in the History of Philosophy*. Oxford, Clarendon Press, pp. 33–73.

—— (2006). "Deflating Descartes' Causal Axiom." In D. Garber and S, Nadler (eds.), *Oxford Studies in Early Modern Philosophy*, Vol. 3. Oxford, Oxford University Press, pp. 1–31.

Scott, D. (2000). "Occasionalism and Occasional Causation in Descartes's Philosophy." *Journal of the History of Philosophy*, 38, pp. 503–528.

Secada, J. (2000). *Cartesian Metaphysics*. Cambridge, Cambridge University Press.

Sellars, W. (1978). "Berkeley and Descartes: Reflections on the Theory of Ideas." In P. Machamer and R. Turnbull (eds.), *Studies in Perception*. Ohio, Ohio State University Press.

Simmons, A. (1999). "Are Cartesian Sensations Representational?" *Nous*, 33, pp. 347–369.

—— (2001). "Sensible Ends: Latent Teleology in Descartes' Account of Sensation." *Journal of the History of Philosophy*, 39, pp. 49–75.

—— (2003). "Descartes on the Cognitive Structure of Sensory Experience." *Philosophy and Phenomenological Research*, 67, 3, pp. 549–579.

Smith, K. (2005). "Descartes' Ontology of Sensation." *Canadian Journal of Philosophy*, 35, 4, pp. 563–584.

Sterelny, K. (1983). "Natural Kind Terms." *Pacific Philosophical Quarterly*, 64, pp. 110–125.

Tye, M. (2002). "Visual Qualia and Visual Content Revisited." In D. J. Chalmers (ed.), *Philosophy of Mind*. Oxford, Oxford University Press, pp. 447–456.

Vinci, T. (1998). *Cartesian Truth*. Oxford, Oxford University Press.

—— (2005). "Reason, Imagination and Mechanism in Descartes' Theory of Perception." In D. Garber and S. Nadler (eds.), *Oxford Studies in Early Modern Philosophy*, Volume II, pp. 35–74.

—— (2008) "Mind–Body Causation, Mind–Body Union and the 'Special Mode of Thinking.'" *British Journal of the History of Philosophy*, 16, 3, pp. 461–488.

Watson, R. (1966). *The Downfall of Cartesianism*, 1673–1712. The Hague, Martinus Nijhoff.

Wee, C. (2006). *Material Falsity and Error in Descartes' Meditations.* London, Routledge.

Wilson, C. (2003). *Descartes's Meditations. An Introduction.* Cambridge, Cambridge University Press.

Wilson, M. (1978). *Descartes.* London, Routledge.

—— (1990). "Descartes on the Representationality of Sensation." In M. Kulstad and J. Covel (eds.), *Central Themes in Early Modern Philosophy.* Indianapolis, Hackett, pp. 1–22. Reprinted in Wilson (1999), pp. 69–83.

—— (1991). "Descartes on the Origin of Sensation." *Philosophical Topics,* 1, 19, pp. 293–323. Reprinted in Wilson (1999), pp. 41–68.

—— (1992). "Descartes on the Perception of Primary Qualities." In S. Voss (ed.), E*ssays on the Philosophy and Science of Rene' Descartes.* Oxford, Oxford University Press, pp. 162–76. Reprinted in Wilson (1999), pp. 26–40.

—— (1999). *Ideas and Mechanism. Essays on Early Modern Philosophy.* Princeton, Princeton University Press.

Yolton, J. (1984). *Perceptual Acquaintance: From Descartes to Reid.* Minneapolis, University of Minnesota Press.

Index